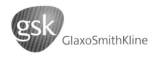

The expression "a picture is worth a thousand words" is particularly appropriate when it refers to medical photographs. Words alone can never create the profound impact of photographs that vividly illustrate diseases a physician might still encounter, as well as those that have already been brought under control.

Today, we no longer consider epidemics of the past as public threats. Yet, with ever-changing global dynamics, physicians must be prepared for the possible return of past scourges. An example is smallpox - shocking but possibly real because of today's new and frightening threats. President Bush recently announced that to protect Americans, the smallpox vaccine will be made available, beginning with the military and health care workers. But preparation begins in many ways, including an understanding and recognition of the physical, mental, and social impact these diseases once had on the population. Medical photography can help us reach that understanding.

GlaxoSmithKline, in its continual effort to serve the public welfare and the medical community, has commissioned an original educational series of four photographic books on the history of medicine from the Burns Archive of Medical Photographic History. These original works, titled "Respiratory Disease: A Photographic History 1845 to 1945," will encourage physicians to think about past medical practices and how medicine has progressed over its most critical century.

This collection, by renowned physician and historian Stanley B. Burns, dominates the field of early medical photography, containing more than 50,000 medically significant photographs. Many of them, complete with written explanations, have never been seen by the general medical profession.

Dr. Burns has published more than a dozen books and his collection has been the subject of numerous exhibitions. Recent presentations have been mounted at the Musee d'Orsay, Paris; Kulturbro 2002 Art Biennial, Brosarp, Sweden; The Center for The Study of the United States, Haifa, Israel; and the National Arts Club, New York. Dr. Burns' full collection of over 700,000 photographs are used by researchers, book publishers, media and film companies worldwide.

GSK is proud to sponsor this original Historical Medical Educational Series.

Chris Viehbacher
President, US Pharmaceuticals
GlaxoSmithKline

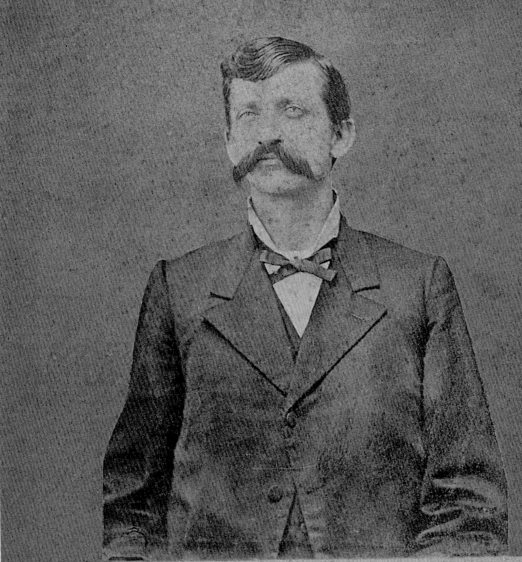

*J. S. Jordan, M. D.*

THROAT AND LUNG PHYSICIAN.

# THE AUTHOR OF THE LUNG RENOVATOR, THE GREAT LUNG REMEDY.

# RESPIRATORY DISEASE:

## A PHOTOGRAPHIC HISTORY
## 1871-1895 THE ANTISEPTIC ERA
### SELECTIONS FROM *THE BURNS ARCHIVE*

STANLEY B. BURNS, M.D.

BURNS ARCHIVE PRESS
NEW YORK 2003

# Colophon

This first edition of *Respiratory Disease: A Photographic History, 1871-1895 The Antiseptic Era* is limited to 20,150 copies including a special cased edition of 1000 copies. The photographs are copyright Stanley B. Burns, MD & The Burns Archive. The design is copyright Elizabeth A. Burns & The Burns Archive.The text and contents of this volume are copyright Stanley B. Burns, MD, 2003. Printed and bound in China for The Burns Archive Press, NY, a division of Burns Archive Photographic Distributors, Ltd. NY. The book is printed on acid free 140 GMS Hi-Q Matte paper. The 4-color separations were scanned at 200 lines per square inch.

ISBN: 0-9612958-5-6

Library of Congress Cataloging-in-Publication Data:
Burns, Stanley B.
*Respiratory Disease: A Photographic History: 1871-1895 The Antiseptic Era*
    Includes bibliographical references: 1. Medical, History
      2. Respiratory Disease  3. Photography, History 4. Lung Disease
      5. Infectious Disease 6. Medical Instruments  7. Stanley B. Burns, MD

## The Burns Archive Press

Author & Publisher: Stanley B. Burns, MD
Editor: Sara Cleary-Burns
Production & Design: Elizabeth A. Burns

## Photographic Captions

**Front Cover: Girl in Plaster of Paris Cast: Treatment for 'Pott's Disease', London, 1877**
Tuberculosis of the spine, also known as "Pott's Disease" or "angular curvature of the spine", caused a typical humpbacked distortion. As the bone tissue was destroyed the spine collapsed, twisted the rib cage and compromised lung volume. Death would follow as pneumonia or tuberculosis exacerbated. Dr. Louis Sayre of Bellevue Hospital, New York, designed a special apparatus to suspend patients while he wrapped his innovative plaster of Paris cast around their bodies. The hardened cast would support the spine. This photograph was taken in London where Dr. Sayre demonstrated his new therapy. In the nineteenth century Europe still dominated the medical field and it was uncommon for American physicians to travel to Europe and educate European doctors.

**Frontispiece: The Great Lung Renovator, Photographic Advertisement, IN, circa 1880**
Physician advertising began as photographic technology improved and the costs reduced. In Terra Haute, Indiana, Dr. J. S. Gordon promoted himself as 'The Developer of The Lung Renovator - The Great Lung Therapy.' Lung disease was the number one killer in the nineteenth century and some physicians capitalized on the public's need for a therapy. Some of the efforts were laudable while others were not.

**Back Cover: Respiratory Physiologist at Work, France, circa 1895**
Laboratory work propelled medicine into the twentieth century. Accurate diagnosis, discovery of the fundamentals of disease, and new therapies all emerged from the laboratory. This physician is studying respiratory physiology. While riding a stationary bicycle the patient breathes into a machine that measures gas exchange. The photographic set up in this image is very primitive. The photographer has simply hung a white cloth as background so the details of the procedure could be recorded. Ironically, it would have been of more benefit to medical historians if the actual work place was visible.

# CONTENTS

PREFACE

THE ANTISEPTIC ERA 1871-1895

LIST OF PHOTOGRAPHS

BIBLIOGRAPHY

PHOTOGRAPHIC TERMS

DEDICATION & ACKNOWLEDGEMENTS

# PREFACE

As an ophthalmologist, a life-long collector and a historian, I am fascinated by our past and drawn to visualizing history. When I first started collecting medical photographs in 1975, I chose images based on both their importance as historic documents and as evidence of medicine's rich past. What I soon realized was their artistic strength.

In 1979, I created the Burns Archive, which is dedicated to preserving medical photographs and producing publications on the history of medical photography. By the mid-1980s, noted curators and artists became interested in medical photography as art. Marvin Heiferman curated "In the Picture of Health" in 1984, an exhibit of more than 140 photographs from the Archive. This was the first exhibition of medical photographs in a public art institution. In 1987, Joel-Peter Witkin edited *Masterpieces of Photography: Selections from the Burns Archive*. Since then, numerous major museums and galleries, recognizing the artistic value of these images, have started to collect and exhibit medical photography. These institutions now display vintage medical photographs of patients, procedures and practitioners to the general public.

What I have learned these past twenty-eight years is that art matters. Art elevates and stimulates us to see things differently. Art creates a different perspective and point of view. When medical photographs are presented to the public, the images are viewed and conceived in terms of personal mortality, human fragility and the vagaries of life. Terror and fascination draw the non-medical public into dialogue with these images. Although the art world's appreciation of vintage medical photography as art is laudable, my original goal as a historian was to present these photographs to my colleagues not as art, but as historic documents. I want my fellow physicians to visually experience the practice of medicine in the 19th century to help them gain a better understanding of the foundation of our therapies and patient treatment. As a physician, I am brought back to a different reality by these photographs. I see my patients; I see difficulties in therapy, I see personal challenges and I wonder whether what I am doing and what I believe in will one day be proven wrong.

GlaxoSmithKline has given me the opportunity to share with my colleagues these photographs on respiratory disease. This compilation is not meant to be an encyclopedic history of the topic, but to put the emphasis on artistic, medical photographs that will allow you to see the transition of medicine from yesterday to today. Many of the treatments depicted have long since become outmoded, but our predecessors believed they were offering the best therapy available. My hope is that you will look at these images as icons of our past and gain a better understanding of what we do and how we can better serve our patients.

Medicine's quest to unselfishly help and heal is one of mankind's highest goals. I am proud to be part of the medical profession and share these photographs to further that goal.

Stanley B. Burns, M.D., F.A.C.S.
New York, March 2003

# The Antiseptic Era 1871-1895

During this time period the final two major medical discoveries, the germ theory of disease and the x-ray, are revealed ending the dark ages of medicine. In 1882, Dr. Robert Koch not only presented the concepts of the germ theory of disease and outlined the procedures necessary to determine the cause of disease but also discovered the bacterial cause of tuberculosis. In December 1895, physicist Conrad Roentgen discovered the x-ray. Koch's discoveries together with the pioneering work of chemists, biologists and physicians laid the groundwork for the field of immunology. In 1890, Dr. Emil von Behring working with Dr. Shibasaburo Kitasato discovered the world's first specific therapy, diphtheria antitoxin. The discovery of a serum based cure for a disease set the direction of immunological research for the next 60 years. The 'Age of Serology' was to last until 1950.

Research laboratory work became the foundation of modern medicine. Scientific based medicine became the accepted norm. Hospitals focused on research and training as well as patient care. In Europe German scientists lead the world in discoveries and research. In America in the 1890s Dr. William Welch, and a group of medical educational pioneers established the Johns Hopkins Hospital resident system that would become the template for medical education world wide in the twentieth century.

Slowly the principles of antiseptic surgery were accepted as a necessary standard. As with many medical innovations it took time for the older practitioners to give up their antiquated ways. It was not until the mid-1880s, almost 20 years after the discovery, that antiseptic surgery was generally accepted. Antiseptic and aseptic surgical methods allowed the development of previously forbidden procedures. An old Latin proverb translated as 'Do Not Enter Here' had been the medical dictum for surgery on the brain, abdomen, neck and chest but this all changed by 1895 and surgical pioneers were devising life saving procedures and safely invading these organs.

Several medical specialties were firmly established. Otologists and laryngologists devised and improved instruments and procedures for better diagnosis and treatment. Thoracic surgeons refined methods for the introduction of medication into the lungs. Sanitary and public health measures were instituted and developed into an important aspect for control of respiratory and intestinal tract diseases.

While respiratory disease remained the number one killer of both children and adults in this era, new therapies, surgical procedures and public health measures would soon achieve a decline in these dreaded scourges. These photographs of practitioners, innovators, procedures and patients represent important facets of this transitional time in medicine.

1

## Nasal Lavage

### Tintype, 2 1/2 by 4 1/2 inches
### circa 1872

Treatment of nasal and upper respiratory tract infection was of prime importance in the pre-antibiotic era. One time honored and safe therapy was a simple irrigation of the infected area. The addition of a therapeutic agent assisted in this treatment. The device being demonstrated is a 'Nasal Douche', which was advertised for routine "cleansing and medicating the nasal passages". It also claimed to help clear the necrotic debris typically left by the ravages of syphilis and tuberculosis. Passing irrigating fluid into one nostril allowed this fluid to flow through the septum into the other nostril and out. Each side was alternately cleansed. Nasal lavage using a variety of powerful chemicals continued as a treatment well into the twentieth century. In 1926, master rhinologist, Arthur W. Proetz, M.D. (1888-1966), published his classic studies on the nose. He stated the action of nasal cilia was important to good health and many traditional therapies actually inhibited ciliary movement and harmed normal debridement. He also recommended the use of isotonic saline solutions infused with a bulb syringe, a treatment still used today. The discovery of antibiotics dramatically cured almost all of the bacterial infections, which required such drastic treatments and ended not only routine nasal levage as a therapy but many of the operations that had been performed on the mastoid, ear and nasal passages. This photograph was probably used to convince patients how safe and easy it was to cleanse the nose.

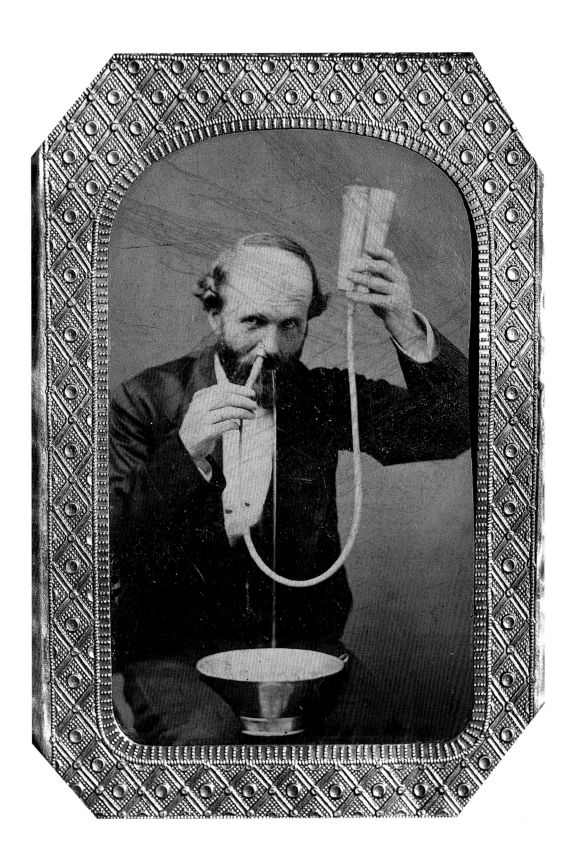

## 2
## Physician with an Oxygen Tank and Special Delivery Apparatus

"Miss Libby," Photographer
Norway, Maine
Cabinet Card
circa 1875

The administration of oxygen was one of the few effective nineteenth century therapies for lung disease. While oxygen did not cure disease it provided relief for respiratory distress common in tuberculosis, asthma, or pneumonia. There were no specific therapies for these diseases. Although oxygen was recognized very early as an important adjunct in treating lung disease, the oxygen tent and aggressive respiratory therapies were not routinely utilized until the second and third decades of the twentieth century. This physician poses beside an oxygen tank holding the gas delivery apparatus. The tank label denotes 1870 as the year of patent and production. Gas therapy in various forms had been popular since the late eighteenth century. This photograph most likely documents the doctor's invention of this particular delivery device.

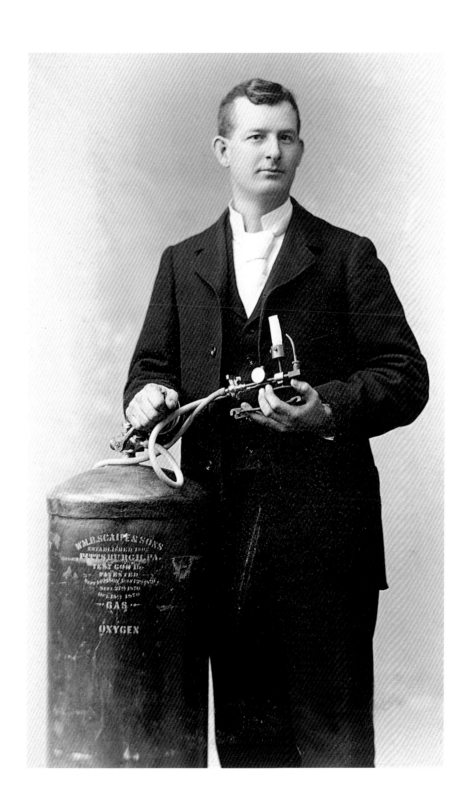

## 3
## 'Pott's Disease' Tuberculosis of the Spine in a Ten Year Old Girl
### Woodburytype, 3 by 4 inches
### London
### 1877

Although it is primarily a lung affliction, tuberculosis can attack every organ system of the body. One complication, tuberculosis of the spine, was also known as Pott's Disease, gibbus or tuberculosis spondylitis. In many cases it caused the spinal column to twist and collapse. This distorted spine compressed the ribs, which drastically reduced the air capacity of the lungs together with the patient's ability to breathe easily. The reduced lung volume and ventilation set the stage for either advanced pulmonary tuberculosis or simple pneumonia. The pain associated with this collapse was significant and also hindered respiration. New York orthopedic surgeon, Lewis Albert Sayre (1820-1900), 'the father of American orthopedic surgery', was a noted innovator. He designed an inventive treatment for Pott's disease and lateral curvature of the spine. Sayre suspended his patient from a large tripod device and then applied plaster of Paris to create a body cast. With the spine supported by the cast the pain was relieved by reducing spine and lung compression. This gave the body a chance to heal (see cover photograph). Dr. Sayre was one of the few Americans invited to Europe to demonstrate medical technique. Throughout the nineteenth century European physicians were the world's leaders. Americans usually traveled to Europe to study medicine and learn new techniques and therapies or invited European physicians to American institutions. When Dr. J.C. Gooding of Cheltenham learned of Dr. Sayre's miracle treatment, he asked Sayre to treat his ten year old daughter, Mabel. Since 19 months of age she had been afflicted with Pott's disease of the cervical and upper dorsal vertebrae. The child suffered from partial paraplegia and the progressive increase of both pain and deformity. "She could not stand or walk without supporting herself on some article of furniture." On examination Dr. Sayre noted, "the pain was so great upon the slightest touch of her back that I feared any attempt to apply the jacket would be useless." But the little girl begged Dr. Sayre to try. He agreed and fixed his suspension tripod "over the mother's chair (the child was lying in her lap), and after carefully adjusting the head rest and auxiliary straps, so as to make the tension even. I pulled her up very slowly from her mother's lap, telling her all the time to let me know if she had the least pain anywhere (as I should have then stopped). She made no complaint whatever but on the contrary, seemed very much pleased, and in a few minutes she was completely lifted from her mothers lap. As she swung off, and was entirely suspended by the head and axillae, she almost instantly exclaimed, 'Mamma, that is so comfortable.'" After finding the suspension had relieved the child's pain, on July 25, 1877, Dr. Sayre applied a plaster of Paris cast to the patient at London's Guy's Hospital in front of an audience 'of the most distinguished surgeons of London.' The child soon learned to walk unsupported and was relatively free of pain. This cast was again changed on August 4th to an improved version (see front cover). Dr. Gooding wrote Sayre, "The child's breathing has been deeper, a fact independently noticed by her mother and myself. And there is certainly more colour in her hitherto pale cheek." In 1878, Dr. Sayre published this and 21 other photographs in his text on treating spinal curvature. Dr. Sayre's technique became the standard treatment for spinal curvatures and, although modernized, his plaster of Paris dressing remains in use to this day.

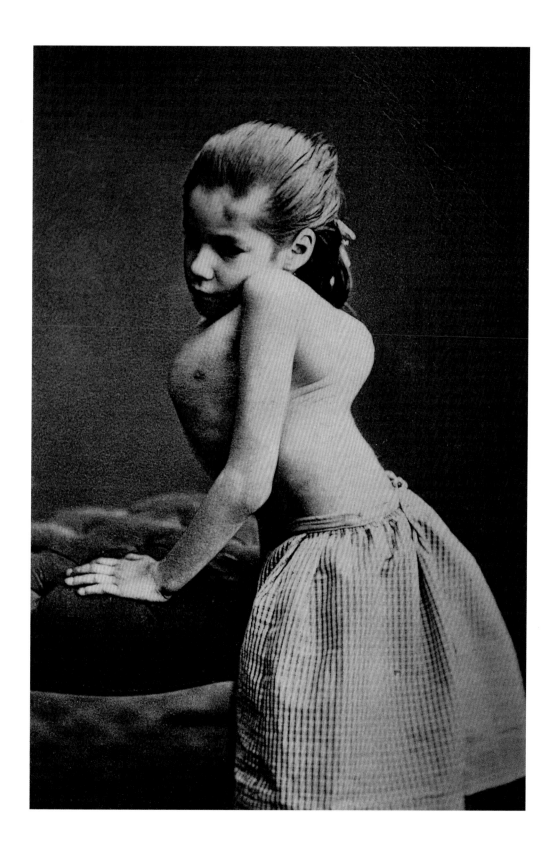

4

## Parotid Tumor Resection: Pre and Post Op Result

James Robinson, DDS, Photographer
Cabinet Card
Dublin, Ireland
circa 1876

In the early years of photography head and neck lesions were the most frequently photographed diseases. The parotid gland and other facial tumors were favored medical subjects especially when the surgeon could document his pre and post-operative results. Social acceptance was dependent on one's visual presentation to the world. It was important that surgeons develop operations that would eliminate deformity. Until the end of the nineteenth century the chest, brain and abdomen were generally off limits to surgeons and operated upon only in the direst of circumstances. Head and neck surgery and limb amputations did not have the constraints of exposure demanded by internal operations. This photograph taken by Dr. James Robinson, dental-surgeon turned-photographer, is from a series taken for surgeons in Dublin, Ireland. The photographs were published as engravings accompanying case reports in the *Dublin Journal of the Medical Sciences*.

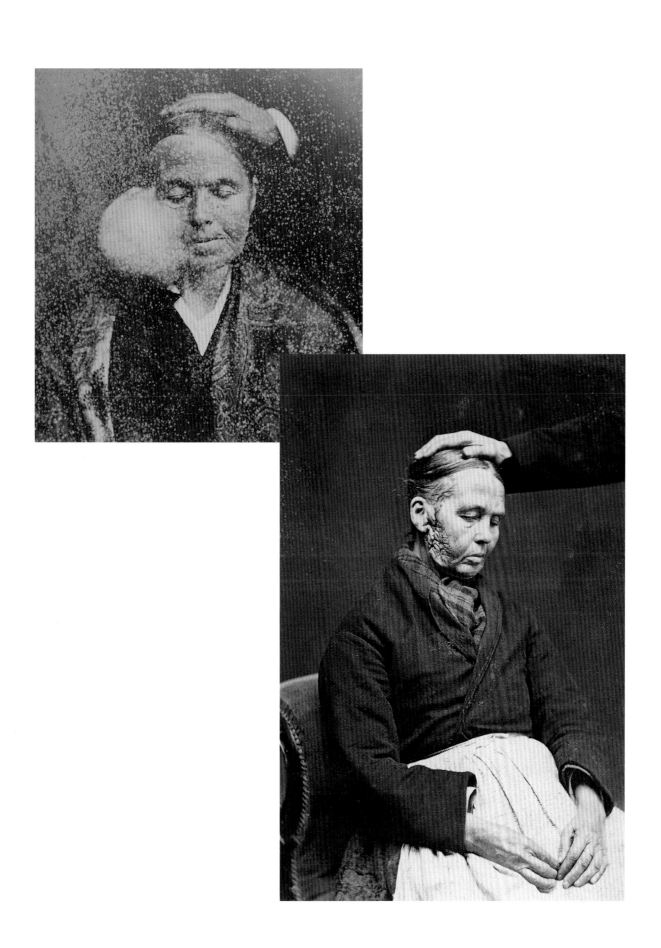

# The Clothes Collectors: London Epidemic Sanitary Workers

## John Thomson, photographer
## Woodburytype, 5 by 5 inches
## London
## 1877

The industrial revolution and immigration brought millions of people into cities. Intestinal and respiratory diseases were rampant for a multitude of reasons: poor sanitation, little or no refuse removal, contaminated and inadequate water supplies, deficient heat in the winter, poor diets, and, especially, the extremely crowded living conditions in poorly ventilated buildings. Epidemics often killed thousands. In 1842, Edwin Chadwick, a lawyer, published a study, which demonstrated that communicable disease was associated with filthy environmental conditions. Disease was now considered an enemy of the entire community, not merely an eye-averting characteristic of the poor. The English pioneer epidemiologist, William Budd, M.D. (1811-1880), discovered in 1856 typhoid, like cholera, was a waterborne disease. He advocated general disinfecting as a means of preventing the spread of all diseases. Although it took until 1875 to create an effective Public Health Act, which included the General Board of Health, once in place conditions were radically improved.

This 'disinfection' cart with its supervised sanitary workers was documented shortly following the implementation of the Public Health Act. The white garb was introduced in this era as a symbol of the 'clean' and sanitary uniform. Typhoid fever and other intestinal diseases were dramatically reduced with the improved sanitation and clean water supply. Respiratory disease remained a scourge of crowded living conditions. These could not be so easily ameliorated. One of the awkward but indispensable tasks of these men was to remove all infected clothes, bedding, and personal effects from the victims of typhoid and other diseases. The workers then were required to promptly sterilize the contaminated belongings in ovens specially designed for this purpose. John Thomson published his photographic work in 1877 titled *Street Life in London*. In this landmark book Thompson, the first social photographer, graphically captured the plight of the urban poor. Society could no longer ignore this terrible reality. Tuberculosis and infectious respiratory disease remained an aspect of crowded living conditions until the twentieth century.

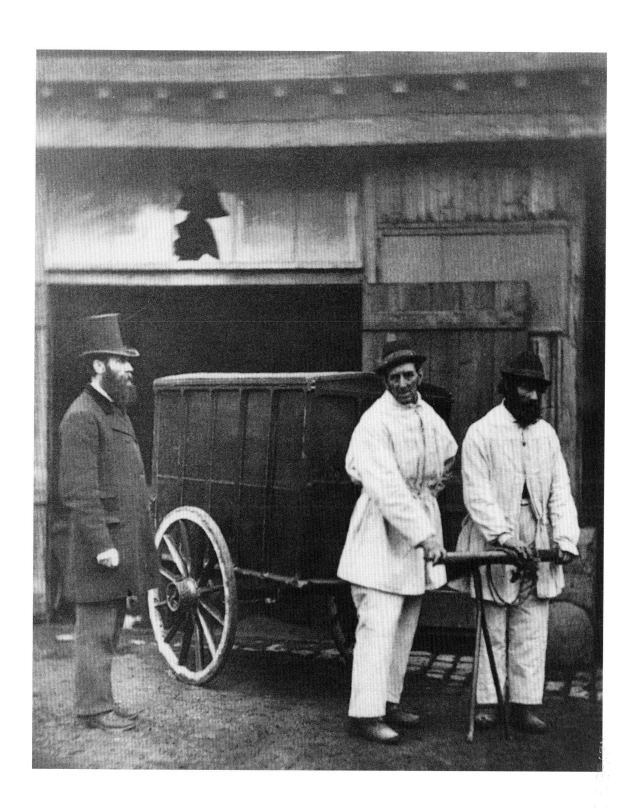

# 6
## First Clinical Photographs of Polio
### The Work of Neurologist, Jean Martin Charcot, MD
### Albumen Print, 3 by 4 inches
### Paris
### circa 1871

Respiratory paralysis and death were a well known facets of polio epidemics in America during the first half of the twentieth century. Though known since ancient times, polio only became epidemic in the last century after the improvement of sanitation. One possible conclusion could be the development of a more pathologic viral strain spread by a fecal-oral route. Exposure to the virus creates a life long immunity to viruses of the same type. Prior to the employment of proper sanitation it has been hypothesized that the disease was so widespread that infants contracted it while still protected by maternal antibodies. The infants not only manifested minimal symptoms and gained life long immunity, but could similarly pass this immunity on. Once sanitation improved, the public educated, and contaminated fecal sources cleaned up, within a generation, a susceptible population evolved. This generation had not contracted the disease and could not pass on protective antibodies. The first major polio epidemic was in New York City in 1916. Prior to that only sporadic cases or small local outbreaks had occurred. There were over 9,000 cases in the New York epidemic and almost all those inflicted were under the age of five. Infantile paralysis was certainly an appropriate name. In the 1930s, the disease began to spread to adults and its name was shortened to polio. During the twentieth century the disease crippled millions, but the associated respiratory paralysis was what killed thousands. The development of positive and negative pressure respiration devices helped preserve some of those with respiratory paralysis. In the 1950s the development of polio vaccines eradicated the scourge in western countries. This is the first published clinical photograph of infantile paralysis. It was commissioned by the world's leading neurologist at that time, Parisian, Jean Martin Charcot, M.D. (1825-1893). Charcot did important pioneer work in polio. Collaborating with Alexander Joffrey, M.D. (1844-1908), he found the prime lesion in polio was the atrophy of the spinal cord's anterior horn cells. Charcot was an advocate of the use of photography in medical publications and the author or editor of several photographic texts and journals. The photographs were taken by Dr. A. Montmeja, a Parisian physician turned medical photographer.

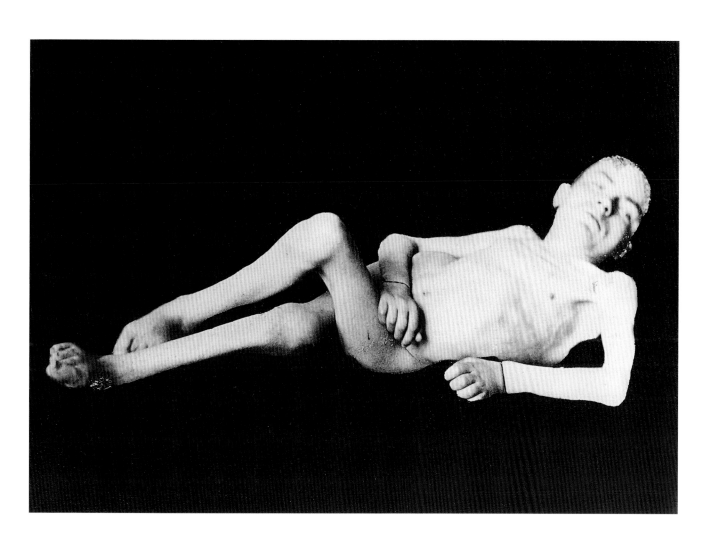

## 7
## DISSECTION PHOTOGRAPHY
## AN INITIATION RITE OF MEDICINE: 'IT'S ALL OVER NOW'
### ALBUMEN PRINT, 5 BY 8 INCHES
### CIRCA 1890

During the nineteenth and throughout the first half of the twentieth century having a photographic portrait taken with one's dissection cadaver became an initiation rite of medicine. The knowledge of anatomy separated physicians from laypersons and the photographs provided evidence of the student's entrance into the profession. Human dissection has been interpreted for centuries in paintings and prints. Rembrandt's *The Anatomy Lesson* and the prints of master anatomists of the 17th and 18th century have become lasting symbols of serious medical study. With the advent of photography, medical students continued the custom. During each decade the composition and posing would change. It became popular to write slogans on the dissection table in about 1890. In this era the oiled cloth lab coats were often inscribed with various handwritten comments. The wide cross section of home states and fraternity letters on these gowns suggest this photograph was taken at a medical school of some importance in a large, Eastern city. It was not until the early 1880s that dissection became legal in most states, a result of an outrageous grave robbing incident. In 1879, the body of former United States Senator, John Scott Harrison, was stolen and shipped to The Medical College of Ohio, in Cincinnati. He was the son of President William Henry Harrison (1841), and the father of Senator and President-to-be, Benjamin Harrison (1888). The national uproar instigated by his son, brought liberal changes in the dissection laws. Prior to that time in many states only the bodies of condemned criminals were legally available for dissection. Grave robbing was the response to the shortage of cadavers needed to teach medical students. After dissection became legal, dissection photography evolved into a type of 'occupational photograph', which was taken by almost all medical students. The privacy concerns of the later twentieth century ended this practice. In some medical institutions dissecting cadavers has been ended. Students learning from computerized devices and mannequins.

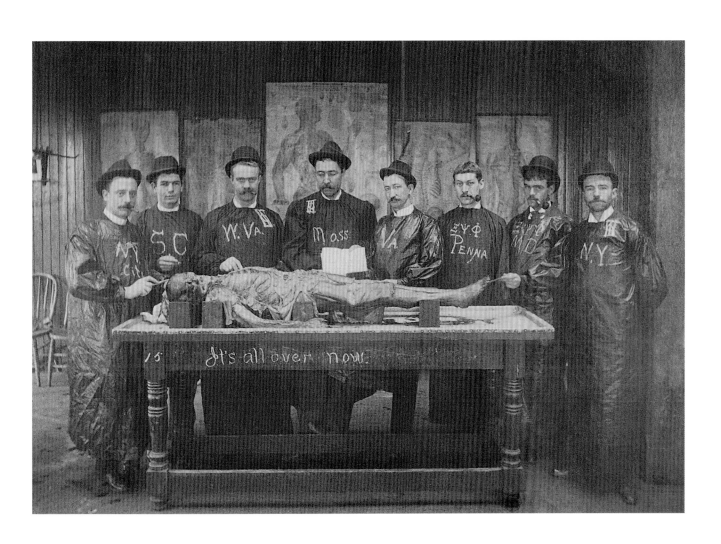

## 8
## Orbital Abscess with Displacement of the Eye

A.H. Geyer, Photographer
Photograuve, 4 by 5 inches
Glasgow, Scotland
1893

Orbital abscess can occur from upper respiratory tract infectious disease. It is a complication that presents with an acute life threatening situation. This abscess has sufficient pus to dramatically displace the patient's eye. In the pre-antibiotic era among the most frequent causes were infections of the respiratory tract that resulted in sinusitis. This patient was treated by incision and drainage of the pus filled mass and, luckily, survived. Unfortunately he lost the vision in the eye.

The eye is protected in a bony socket with little room for pus or tumor tissue hence it is easily forced from its socket. As the eye is attached to the brain via the optic nerve, infection can easily spread along this nerve fiber resulting in encephalitis. The internal apex of the eye socket is in proximity to major brain vessels therefore extension of the infection through the orbital apex results in cavernous sinus thrombosis. As the main vein plexus draining the brain clogs up from the inflammatory process severe cerebral congestion, infection and death occurs. Mastoiditis, sinusitis, and otitis media were so common in the nineteenth century that they were believed by many to be 'normal' conditions. Much like dental cavities were a 'normal' condition in the twentieth century. Normal and healthy are two separate matters. The complications of these 'normal' upper respiratory tract infections were serious and now have, thanks to antibiotics, become rare. Even today, however, an orbital abscess is a life threatening state.

A. Maitland, M.D., who worked at the Charlotte Street Branch of the Glasgow Eye Clinic had his patients photographed. In 1898, he published the images in *Atlas of External Diseases of the Eye*. It was the first photographic atlas of external ophthalmic disease. The photograuves were made by the noted firm of T. & R. Annon. Photography allowed physicians to accurately present their unusual cases. Publications permitted the widest range of dissemination of the images. The 1890s was an era in the production of numerous medical photographic atlases in a wide range of specialties.

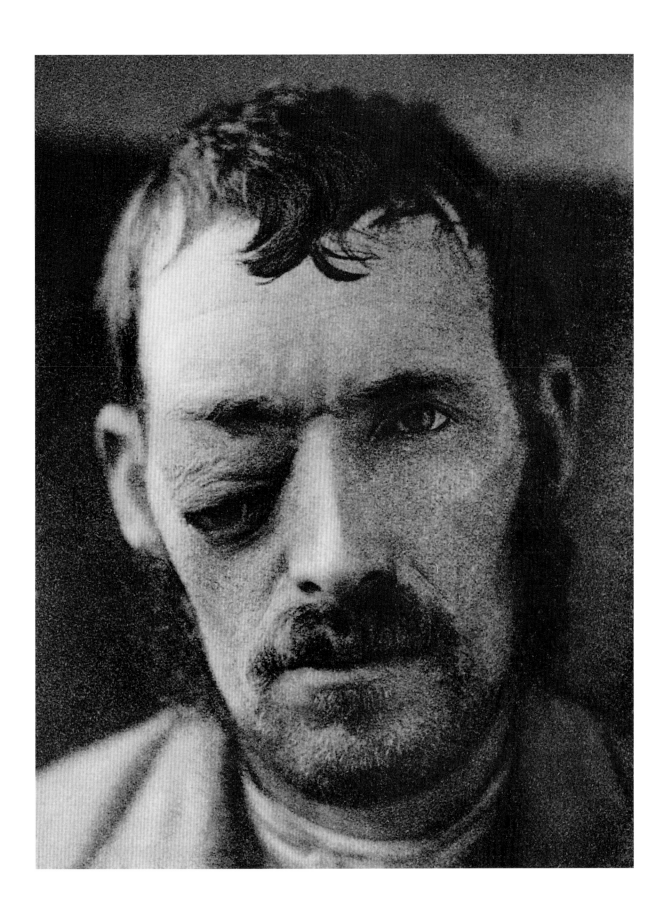

# FATAL SCARLET FEVER COMPLICATION: ELEPHANTIASIS WITH SEPSIS

## O.G. MASON, PHOTOGRAPHER
## ALBUMEN PRINT, 3 BY 4
## BELLEVUE HOSPITAL, NEW YORK
## 1878

Scarlet fever is primarily a local infection of the throat caused by group A hemolytic streptococci. Like other infections caused by this group of streptococci, a soluble toxin is produced. The disease is spread by contact with respiratory tract discharges from the mouth and nose, primarily by hand contact, coughing, sneezing, etc. A variety of symptoms occur dependent on the virulence of the strain causing the infection and the patient's level of immunity. Sore throat, fever, headache are followed by a typical rash appearing within a couple of days from the onset. The rash appears on the upper chest and back first. In Caucasians this rash does not usually involve the face. Complications include rheumatic fever, otitis media, meningitis, nephritis, tonsillitis, and anemia. In a rare case severe toxic septic forms can cause a myriad of fatal complications.

Epidemics of scarlet fever which killed thousands of children were common for centuries. In the 1820s, a more virulent strain evolved. Until about 1875 of all the childhood infections scarlet fever was rated the number one killer of children, even eclipsing diphtheria. In the epidemic of 1735, Belknap in his *History of New Hampshire* notes the severity of the death rate, "In the parish of Hampton Falls it raged most violently. Twenty families buried all of their children, one-sixth part of the inhabitants died within thirteen months. In the whole province, not less than 1,000 persons, of whom 900 were under 20 years of age."

This 17 year old girl contracted scarlet fever at age eight. A lymphangitis developed in her legs and over the next nine years she experienced recurrent bouts of inflammation with progressive edema. Her legs grew to these grotesque proportions while her upper body remained normal. Secondary infection with septicemia caused her death five days after this photograph was taken. She was a patient of dermatologist, George Henry Fox, M.D. (1846-1937) at New York's Bellevue Hospital. The photograph was taken by noted hospital photographer, O.G. Mason. Elephantiasis was a result of toxic lymphangitis, is a rare but recognized complication of various septic, non-parasitic infections. In 1923-4, the Drs. George and Gladys Dick identified the bacterial cause of the disease and developed a skin test to determine susceptibility. Within a few decades the sulfonamides and antibiotics made the infection uncommon.

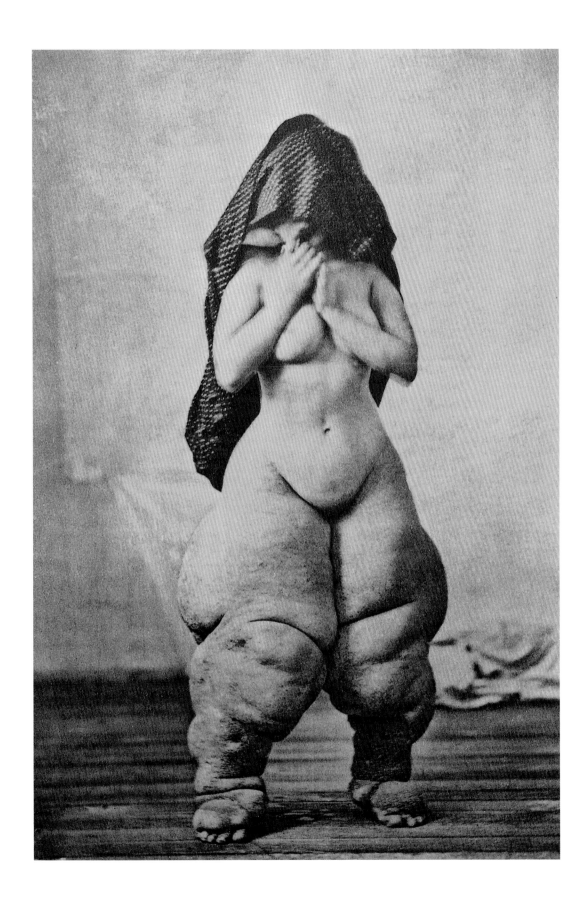

10
## Street Doctor Selling Cough Syrup

John Thomson, Photographer
Woodburytype, 3 by 4 inches
London
1877

The population in a city's poor and immigrant neighborhoods often mistrusted mainstream doctors. They preferred to be treated by self-medication and non-traditional therapies offered by local practitioners or street vendors. Too often the ailment turned out to be tuberculosis. While this nineteenth century scourge cut across all social classes it particularly struck those living in poorly ventilated, cramped city slums. This well dressed street doctor advertises his cough elixir to Londoners in 1877 claiming "Prevention better than Cure". The doctor's high shoes indicate a shortened leg-problem. English social photographer, John Thomson, took this picture for his book on street life in London. Patent medicines appeared to help most patients, as their base was usually alcohol, opium or some other powerful agent.

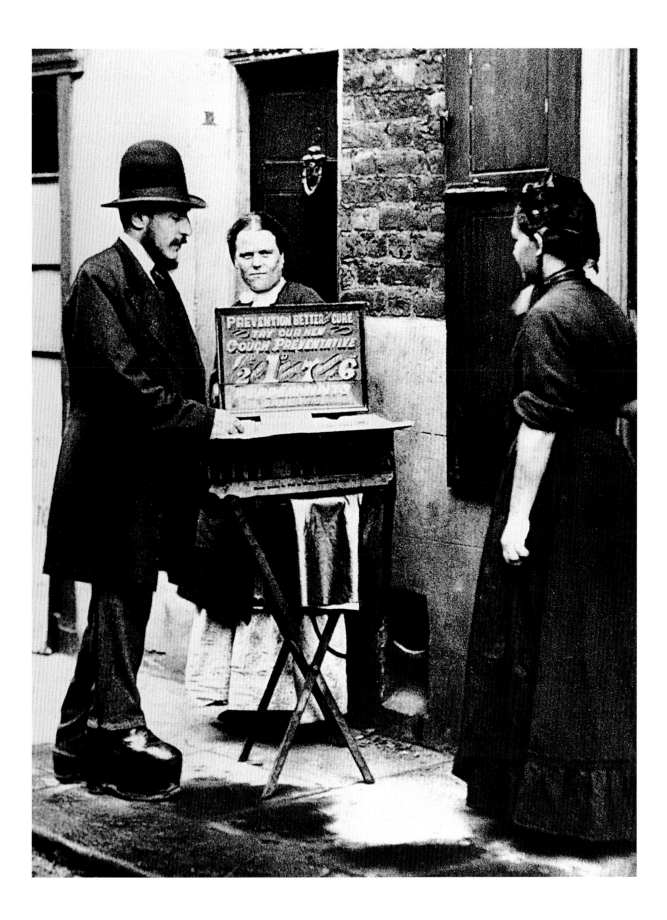

# Eugenicist Francis Galton's Composite Photograph of Consumption

## Woodburytype, 2 by 4 inches
## London
## 1883

This composite photograph from a series taken by eugenicist, Francis Galton, was an attempt to visually identify the individuals who would contract lung disease. He also created a composite specifically for tuberculosis. Galton carried his idea that facial and other body characteristics could identify specific personality types, predict behavior, and even disease states to seeming perfection. He devised the photographic method of 'composite portraiture' to analyze people. At that time the only evidence of heredity available was the physical appearance of individuals. Use of the camera to document and analyze his hypothesis appeared to Galton as a natural progression in his scientific research. He photographed a number of representatives in each group exhibiting identifiable characteristics. He then would superimpose the negatives of the individuals, producing a single composite photograph. A composite image was expected to identify the 'representative type' of each group. Galton asserted the more closely a person resembled a facial a type, the more certain he was to have the other characteristics, such as consumption and tuberculosis.

Francis Galton, the brilliant cousin of Charles Darwin, was a pioneering theoretician and statistician. Unfettered by conventional wisdom, he became a leading figure of nineteenth century science. As well as originating the science of eugenics he was considered the father of bio-statistics. Galton also discovered the individuality of the human fingerprint, contributed to genetics, and developed the anthropometric method, a means used to measure human abilities. It was Galton that advanced the view that inherited characteristics are more important than environmental influences, thus setting in motion the 'nature versus nurture' issue. His eugenics theories on improving the human race by improving the basic human stock gained a major foothold in numerous countries. Hundreds of scientists, as well as social reformers, took up his ideas. Many expanded on his techniques and theories to illustrate or document criminal types and/or undesirables. By 1900, eugenic society movements were active in England, Germany and the United States. In these countries laws were eventually passed regarding sterilization, immigration and a host of related topics. By the 1920s, American county fairs included awards to the 'perfect family.'

This 1883 photograph was published in his landmark book, *Inquiries into Human Faculty and its Development.* Ironically, most of his photographs did not show what he purported. In fact, the irregularities of the subject's features tended to cancel each other out. Consequently, a composite photograph often presented less unusual features than the individual photographs from which it was composed.

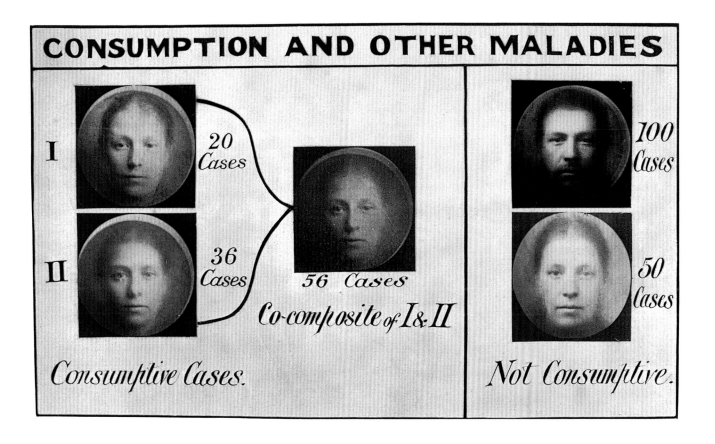

# CONSUMPTION AND OTHER MALADIES

I    20 Cases

II    36 Cases

56 Cases
Co-composite of I & II

Consumptive Cases.

100 Cases

50 Cases

Not Consumptive.

12

## Skundoo, a Chilkat Shaman, Treating a Woman for Tuberculosis

Case and Draper, photographers
Platinum Print, 8 by 10 inches
Juneau, Alaska
1908

This photograph is perhaps the only surviving visual legacy that symbolizes the killing of Native-Americans by pulmonary disease and the treatment provided by their healers. The Chilkat, a branch of the Tlingit tribe, lived on the panhandle of the South Alaskan coast. Most of the Northwest coast tribes, Tlingit, Haida, Kwakiutl, Tsimshian, Nootka and Haisla existed in relative solitude and immunologic isolation until the last third of the nineteenth century. The Yukon and Alaska gold rushes combined with the fishing and timber industries brought the white man and his diseases in unprecedented numbers. Many villages were forced to be abandoned as the native population succumbed in horrifying numbers to the common childhood diseases, small pox and cholera. It is estimated that over 80% of these Native-Americans perished; a population drop from 500,000 to 100,000. Tuberculosis, the number one killer in the nineteenth century, proved to be the final straw completely decimating the surviving population. This rare photograph depicts Skundoo, a well known shaman, treating a woman for tuberculosis whose exposed chest testifies to her disease state. Skundoo has his symbolic paraphernalia consisting of a crown headdress, robes and bone rattle. In the background is a Tlingit pillow and carved poles. These are not totem poles but represent guardian figures associated with the power of the shaman. Tuberculosis triumphed as hundreds of thousands died. Shamans and shamanism eventually disappeared as an important cultural force. It is only with the recent attempt to restore the cultural integrity of the Native American that shamanism has resurfaced. All known historic shaman healing scenes (less than a dozen known) are posed as these healing sessions usually occurred at night in the patient's home. The posed images, however, allow a glimpse into the nature of this healing practice.

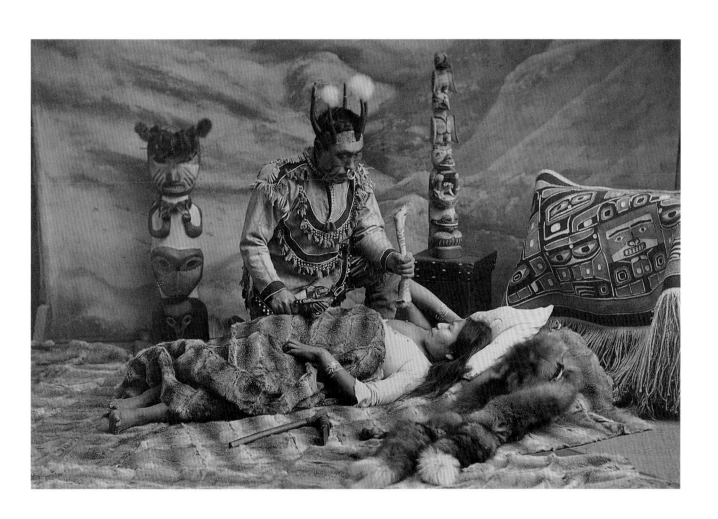

## 13
## Ear, Nose & Throat Hospital Staff
### Gelatin Silver Print, 7 by 9 inches
### Chicago
### circa 1892

The development of specialties such as otolaryngology and ophthalmology gave new status to hospitals and their associated physicians. Not only were separate departments created in established hospitals but entire specialized hospitals were founded by the physicians in these new fields. Until the closing years of the nineteenth century, hospitals were not life saving medical sanctuaries and were avoided by both patients and doctors. They were not only known for the spread of infection but as the final resting place for the dying poor. Association with a hospital was often perceived as bad for one's health and practice. Most physicians worked independently, treating patients in private homes or offices, as well as establishing their own health care facilities. It was both the development of scientific and medical laboratories together with medical specialization that helped secure the professional image of the hospital. The general public was slowly acclimated to the idea that hospital could do more good than harm. By the 1890s, hospital personnel had no qualms about publicly demonstrating their hospital affiliation. This group of specialists, staff of the Homeopathic Hospital's Eye, Ear, Throat, and Nose Clinic in Chicago, are proudly posed on the steps of their clinic. This style of photograph was typical of the era and representative of this change in attitude. Apparently the hospital staff had gathered to celebrate some special occasion as close inspection reveals many of those present are holding ribbon decorated parade bugles; a curious combination of both the serious and frivolous. By the early twentieth century, a physician's hospital association, especially if it was part of a well-known medical school, became the highest mark of his achievement.

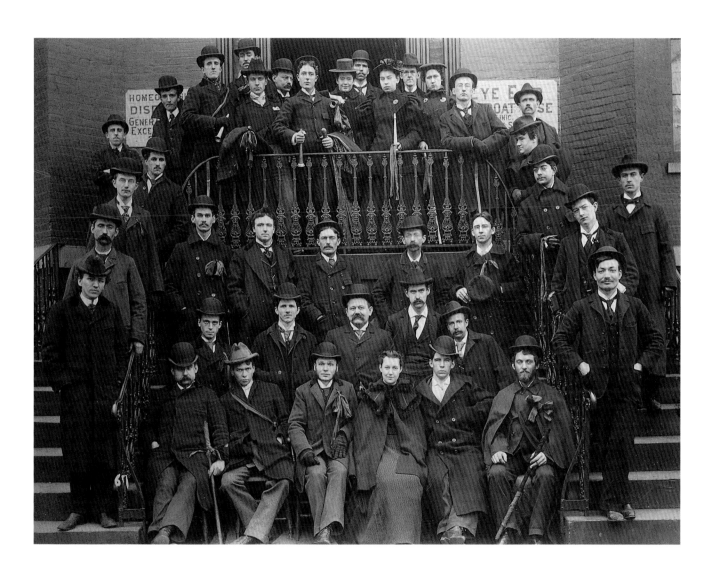

## 14
## Dr. Isaac Abt Supervises Ear, Nose & Throat Clinic

Gelatin Silver Print, 8 by 10 inches
Chicago
circa 1895

Since the late nineteenth century, clinical teaching has given medical students hands-on experience in the art of healing. However, photographs in clinical settings with noted medical personalities are extremely rare from this era. This image of Dr. Isaac Arthur Abt (1867-1955) supervising a resident as he examines a patient's nose provides a wealth of information about early clinics. The photographer has created an assembly-line effect by photographing the two residents with their patients side by side. This angle also visually underscores the limited importance of the student. The bearing and watchful eye of the physician-in-charge, Dr. Abt, is skillfully emphasized by the placement of his assistant in the background. Professor of Diseases of Children at two major Chicago area medical schools, Rush and Northwestern, Dr. Abt played an important role in the establishment of Pediatrics as a specialty. He was president of several national pediatrics societies, editor of pediatric journals and an author of numerous texts. Upper respiratory tract disease was an important aspect in pediatric practice, so it's not too surprising to see Dr. Abt supervising an adult ENT clinic.

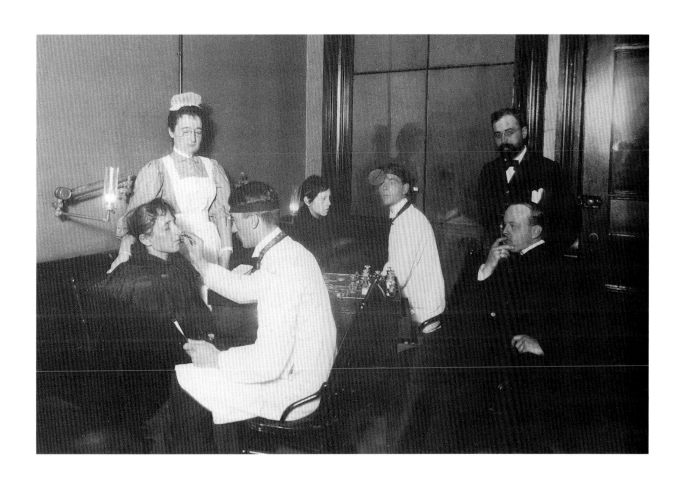

## 15
# WOMAN WITH URTICARIA
## ALBUMEN PRINT, 4 BY 5 INCHES
## PARIS
## CIRCA 1872

This patient presents with skin writing or dermatographism, a bizarre but harmless phenomena that occurs in certain hypersensitive states. Medical photographers in the nineteenth century were fascinated by this phenomenon and numerous artistic photographs exist documenting the condition. This photograph, one of the earliest of this condition, depicts much of the patient's body. As medical diagnostic expertise progressed and physicians were able to accurately focus more and more on the cause of disease, medical photography focused closer and closer to the actual lesion. By the third decade of the twentieth century the patient's identity was secondary and the lesion was primary. Confronting a full view of a patient forces practitioners to deal with the whole patient not just the disease. Today a return to a more holistic approach to patients has become popular.

Urticaria, more commonly known as hives, is a vascular reaction of the skin characterized by the sudden appearance of red and white swelling. The swellings represent localized areas of edema called wheals. These wheals, which are intensely pruritic, rarely last longer than 48 hours. This time frame distinguishes them from other skin lesions. In some patients, they become chronic and recurrent for weeks and sometimes years. Almost any immunology, chemical or physical insult can cause urticaria. Food allergy is the most common immunologic cause of urticaria. Insect bites, pollens, inhalants, ingestants (especially drugs) and infection have also been associated with its onset. Urticaria was given its name from the reaction that occurs when the skin is touched by the plant known as urtica, or stinging nettle. 'Urticaria, or nettle-rash, is thought to be caused by the minute hairs or prickles of the urtica plant which transmits a venomous fluid when pressed.

Since the advent of antibiotics and the conquest of many respiratory infections that plagued mankind, allergic respiratory conditions have become increasingly important. Air pollution and air borne allergens have substantially added to the respiratory system's allergic response. Asthma and emphysema have increased to alarming proportions in many communities and become a major public health concern.

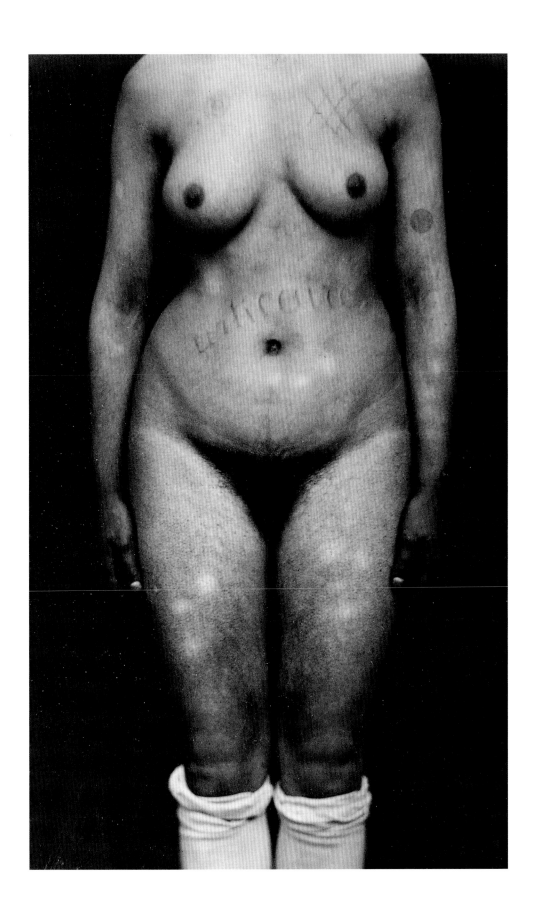

16
## Woman with Black Smallpox Six Hours Before Death

Gelatin Silver Print, 5 by 7 inches
New York City
1881

Most physicians know the skin eruptions and 30% mortality rate of smallpox, but few are aware of a previously 100% fatal form of the disease, 'black smallpox.' This virulent form of the disease often attacks the lungs and other internal organs, causing extreme toxemia and hemorrhage, which kills the patient a few days before the classic skin eruptions would have appeared. These patients have only a slight, nondescript red rash. The usual cause of death in smallpox, in the classic condition, was secondary bacterial infection, which presented in the massive skin eruptions. Several other fatal complications, however, could also develop. In black smallpox, the pox was internal. These patients died from hemorrhage in the lungs or intestinal tract. They essentially drown in their own blood from corroding internal lesions in the respiratory tract, especially lung lesions. In the toxic form, the blood clotting mechanism was also upset which caused additional internal hemorrhage. The name, black smallpox, came from the color of crusted blood about the body orifices and the black bowel movements that were due to internal bleeding. This woman, a victim of the 1881 smallpox outbreak in New York City, was photographed at an isolated smallpox hospital located on an island in the East River. Caked, dark colored blood is evident on the woman's nostrils and mouth. This is the earliest known photograph of the deadly condition.

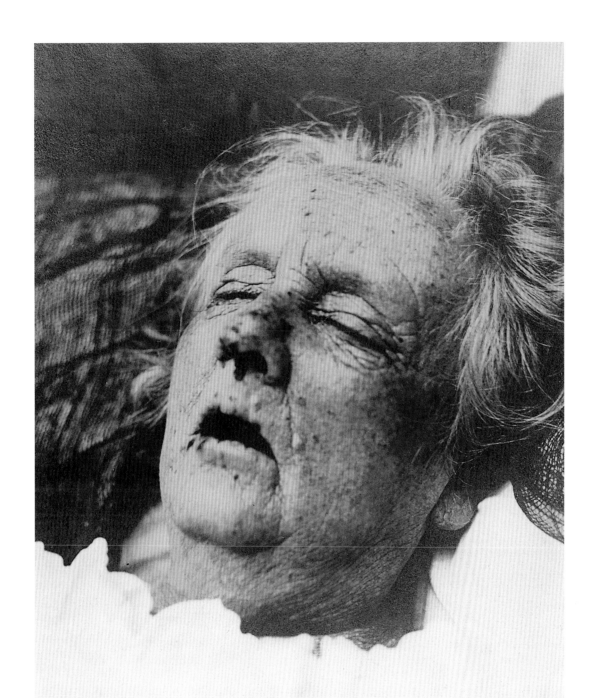

Black Smallpox, without eruption
6 hours before death.

## 17
## President Ulysses S. Grant
## Three Days Before Death from Throat Cancer

### U.S. Instantaneous Photographic Company
### Gelatin Silver Print, 10 by 13 inches
### New York
### July 20th, 1885

One of Americans most beloved presidents, Ulysses S. Grant, was admired for his critical role in winning the Civil War. As president, he oversaw reconstruction and tried to keep an even hand in his dealings, while still assisting the African Americans. As Grant dictated to his secretary, he began to feel pain in his throat, which soon made eating almost impossible. Grant was diagnosed with fatal throat cancer on November 1, 1884. Grant, a New Yorker, retired to his country home in Mount McGregor located in the Adirondack Mountains. The president's last days were recorded by photographers and issued as a set of souvenir photographs. His funeral procession down Fifth Avenue was the largest ever held in New York.

Grant wasn't only the only president diagnosed with cancer in the head area. In 1893, President Grover Cleveland developed cancer of the jaw. His operation took place on a yacht in Long Island Sound and was performed by one of Philadelphia's leading surgeons, W.W. Keen, President Cleveland's operation was successful in two areas; the disease never recurred and the operation was kept secret during a critical time of the nation's financial recovery. In those days privacy was the order of the day for national leaders. A crisis had already swept the nation with the enactment of the Sherman Silver Purchase Act of 1890. Any news of cancer inflicting the president would have caused severe economic repercussions. By the turn of the century, however, the successful result was known and stereoview cards were issued showing the operating room. In 1917, Dr. Keen told the complete story of the operation. Some of President Cleveland's tissue had been deposited in the Mutter Museum. Reexamined in 1976 with modern pathologic knowledge and techniques the tumor was found to be a non-metastatic type of cancer. It was a verrucous carcinoma associated with the human papillomatous virus. Cleveland died June 24, 1908 in Princeton, New Jersey of heart failure following complications of pulmonary thrombosis and edema.

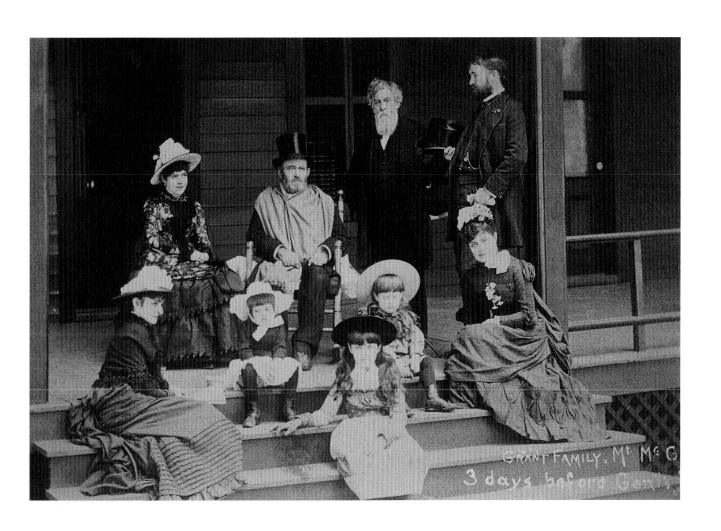

GRANT FAMILY. Mt McG

3 days before Gen.

## 18
## Electro Therapy for Throat Disease
### Photograuve, 3 by 4 inches
### circa 1890

Electrical delivery devises used for medical treatment, diagnosis, research and therapy, were considered miracles of the era much like the laser of today. In one instance it was proved to be true. Through electrical studies of cathode ray tubes and other physical apparatus the x-ray was developed. Physiologists had demonstrated that electricity was a basic phenomenon of the life process. Pioneer French neurologist, Duchenne de Bolougne, used electricity to show neural and muscular activity, evidencing further use and importance of electricity in the normal and disease state. During the 1860s and 70s a multitude of machinery was developed to deliver electricity in various forms. In this photograph a large static charge machine is being used to treat a patient's throat disease. Almost every throat condition from cancer to allergy was treated by various electrical charges. During its time the static machine procedure was quite an impressive technique and patients, as well as physicians, believed they were involved in the most advanced techniques in medical therapy. Ultimately the lack of clinical response resulted in the demise of the electrotherapeutic machines. Electro-cautery used in surgery, and electric implants and treatments for pain relief, are two important remnants remaining of the electro therapy era.

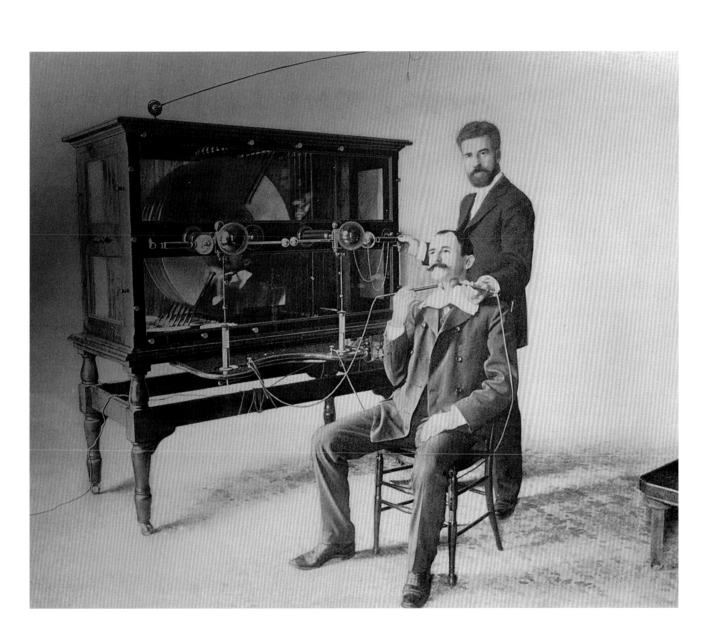

# Doctors on Rounds on Tuberculosis Ward, Bellevue Hospital

## O.G. Mason, Photographer
### Gelatin Silver Print 9 by 12 inches
### New York
### circa 1888

This photograph of house physicians on rounds in the tuberculosis ward at Bellevue Hospital in the 1880s is typical of the effort taken to help change the image of the safety of hospitalization. These large, framed photographs of operating rooms, laboratories and wards were hung in the reception areas and halls. Visitors and patients could then visualize the facilities. Until the last decade of the nineteenth century hospitals had the reputation as places where one went to die. This image was taken by America's most noted hospital photographer, O. G. Mason. He was one of the few photographers that was employed and worked solely in a hospital.

Historic photographs serve to augment written history by providing records of mundane activity that would not normally be recorded. This photograph shows a ward nurse accompanied the physicians on their rounds. It was her job to hold a paper over the face of the tuberculosis patients so the physician could auscultate the chest without fear of air borne particle contamination. This is the earliest known photograph of this concern for particulate contamination. This concern is not seen in European medical photography until the twentieth century. The binaural stethoscope with its long tubing also helped distance the physician from the patient. All of the physicians seen here use a binaural stethoscope but in Europe, the monaural stethoscope, a tube about seven or eight inches long, was the preferred instrument even though it required intimate patient contact.

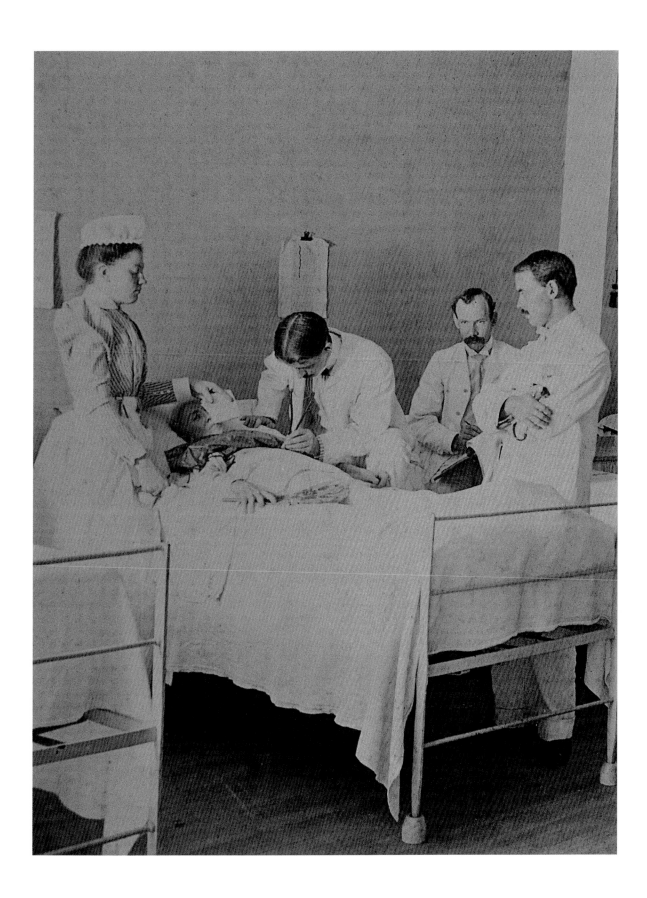

## 20
# The Laboratory: Basis of Modern Medicine

### Gelatin Silver Print, 3 by 5 inches
### France
### circa 1895

It was the development of laboratory based medicine that was the core of modern medical practice and diagnosis. By making possible the positive identification of the disease process, the scientific and clinical laboratories pulled medicine out of the Dark Ages of diagnosis and therapeutics. The work of Robert Koch, M.D. (1843-1910) was particularly important. He firmly established the science of bacteriology and the necessity of the laboratory. In 1877, with his demonstration of the life cycle of the anthrax bacillus Koch was the first to show a specific micro-organism caused a specific disease. The practice of medicine was changed forever with his elucidation in 1882 of the germ theory of disease together with his 'Koch's Postulates' to establish the cause of a disease. Also in 1882, he announced his discovery of the bacterial cause of tuberculosis. For his work in tuberculosis he received the Nobel Prize in Medicine in 1905. While there were dozens of university hospital laboratories studying disease Koch's demonstration proved the laboratories were critical to diagnosis and they soon became a necessary part of every hospital. The universities laboratories remained important research centers and special institutes were established to conduct research. During the next 30 years, the causes of dozens of diseases were discovered. This is a photograph of a hospital laboratory where bacterial and hematological studies were conducted. This is the typical format for the photographs taken of hospital laboratories: A white coated lab director overseeing his technicians. Thousands of such photographs are extent.

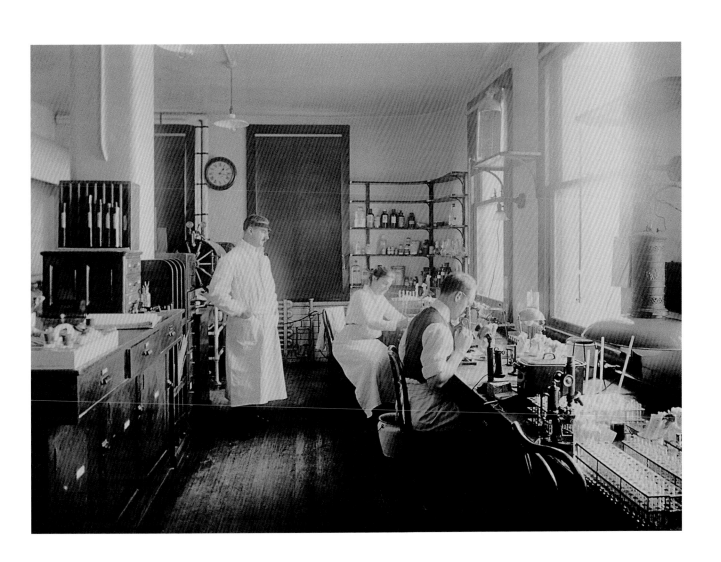

## 21
## Gangrene of the Legs as a Complication of Diphtheria
### Gelatin Silver Print, 5 by 7 inches
### circa 1892

One of the most deadly of childhood's respiratory tract infections was diphtheria. Diphtheria is a local infection of the throat by *Corynebacterium diphtheriae*. It produces a classic odoriferous membrane of the pharynx, tonsils, or palate that can quickly kill its young victims. The odor and an acute swelling of the neck, called 'bull neck', due to rapid lymph node involvement, helps astute physicians to differentiate between diphtheria, streptococcal sore throat, croup or other throat infections. Virulent strains of this bacteria occurred in epidemic form with a mortality of 30 to 50%. While suffocation was the acute life threatening problem the bacteria produced a powerful exotoxin as well that lethally affected distant organ systems. This bacteria does not spread systemically so the primary infection remains in the throat while the exotoxin attacks the heart, central nervous system or other organs. These patients are severely toxic and can have multiple organ system involvement. The peripheral nervous system involvement is peculiar and may be related to the level of toxic effect on the end organ. The characteristic progression in diphtheria is paralysis of the palate, followed by the eyes, muscles, heart, pharynx, larynx and lastly the limbs. This photograph documents a case of diphtheria in which the exotoxin resulted in the rare complication, arteritis, with the end result of gangrene in the legs. Few photographs are extent of patients alive with severe complications of diphtheria as they were extremely toxic and rapidly died.

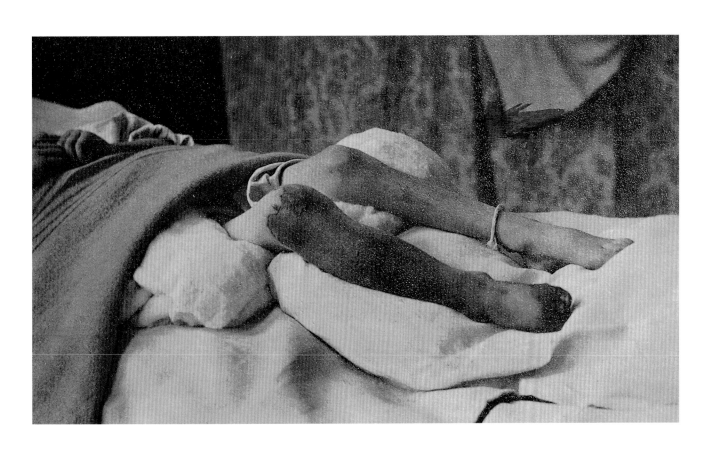

## 22
# EMIL VON BEHRING: DISCOVERER OF DIPHTHERIA ANTITOXIN

### WINNER FIRST NOBEL PRIZE IN MEDICINE, 1901
### PHOTOGRAUVE, 3 BY 4 INCHES
### 1894

The work of Robert Koch, M.D. in bacteriology is rightfully well known. He established the field of accurate diagnosis in the cause of disease. The discoveries of Emil von Behring, M.D. (1854-1917) are less well appreciated today but in 1890, he was the one to develop the world's first specific therapy, diphtheria antitoxin for treatment of the most dreaded of all childhood respiratory diseases, diphtheria. His discovery established the idea that a specific disease could have specific treatment based on immunologic and serum therapies. The next 60 years were known as the 'The Age of Serology', as most workers attempted to find serum based, therapeutic substances such as antitoxins or vaccines, which would cure or prevent disease. Koch's discoveries didn't cure anyone though he had unsuccessfully tried to make a tuberculin serum. Von Behring's did cure. It was thus, Emil von Behring who received the first Nobel Prize in Medicine in 1901. His miracle cure was a proper start for the 20th century. Von Behring not only developed the antitoxin, he created a manufacturing plant for its mass production. By 1894, his antitoxin was saving lives around the world. Immune serum substances were found successful for the treatment of tetanus and serpent poisoning, but were generally unsuccessful in other diseases. It was not the serum and circulating antibodies that would provide the key to therapy but study of the cell itself. In actuality von Behring's success stimulated researchers to emphasize the humeral component of immunity. Cellular immunity study drew comparatively few researchers until the problems of mid-twentieth century allograft rejections. The research shifted from the chemical and chemists to the biologist and study of the cell. The important role of lymphocytes, mast cells and t-cells were soon appreciated. Today it is believed that intracellular DNA holds the key to the conquest of disease.

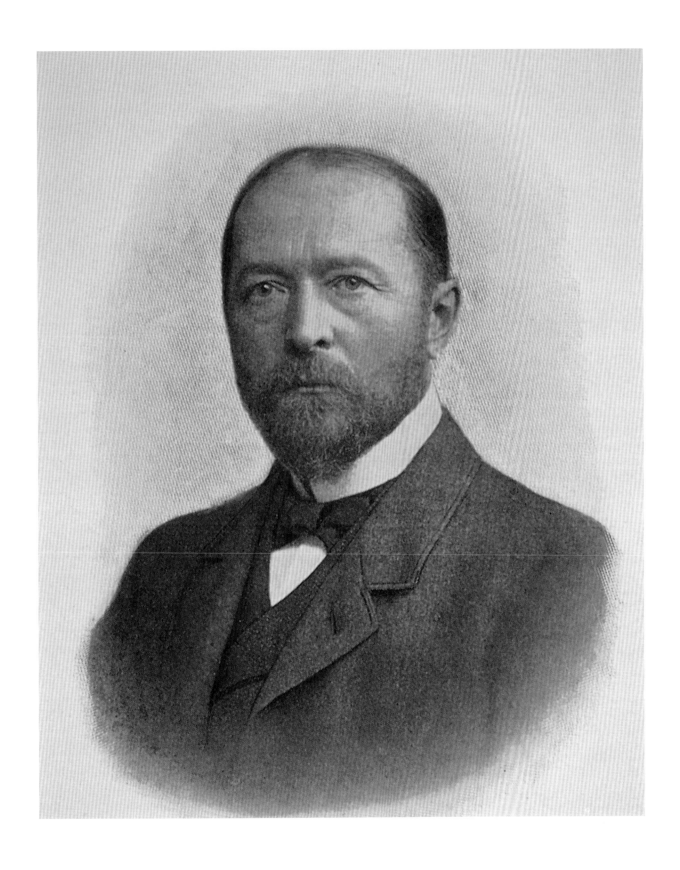

## 23
## DRAINING A MASTOID ABSCESS
### GELATIN SILVER PRINT, 3 BY 5 INCHES
### CIRCA 1895

Infectious upper respiratory tract disease often spread causing inflammation in the ear, sinuses, tonsils, mastoid and other areas. At the turn of the century mastoid, tonsil and adenoid surgery were the most frequent procedures of otolaryngologists. Infections of the mastoid if left untreated could result in death as the infection was spread directly or thru veins into the middle or posterior cranial fossas. This would with result in a brain abscess, meningitis or even prolapse of the brain through an eroded bony defect. At best, middle ear and mastoid infections would leave the patient with decreased hearing or deafness. This impacted speech, learning, as well as social and vocational development. The seriousness of draining ear infections was recognized from the time of Hippocrates but it was not until the sixteenth century that surgical intervention was devised. Parisian surgeon, Jean Petit, in the early 18th century is credited with performing the first successful operation for removing mastoid pus. During the nineteenth century, after the discovery of general anesthesia, mastoid surgery rapidly progressed. In 1873, Hugo Rudolf Schwartze, M.D. of Halle, Germany and James Hinton, M.D. of London, independently, described the simple mastoidectomy procedure. It was the operation of choice in acute mastoiditis but was insufficient to cure chronic mastoiditis. The 'radical mastoidectomy' was an advancement on the Schwartze procedure proposed by German surgeons in 1889. Prior to this development mastoid operations frequently failed because the surgeons waited until the infection was too far advanced. In 1899, Otto Korner, M.D. showed that hearing could be left intact by careful dissection. In 1910, Gustav Bondy, M.D. devised the 'modified radical mastoidectomy', an even less aggressive approach to the mastoid. Operating early was the key to cure. By the 1930s Bondy's operation became the standard. The introduction of the sulfonamides in the 1930s and penicillin in the 1940s resulted in a rapid decline of the need for mastoid surgery. This operation, once the commonest of procedures, became rare. The conquest of mastoiditis placed new emphasis on preservation of hearing and otolaryngologists began concentrating on procedures to improve hearing. This photograph shows physicians treating a mastoid infection.

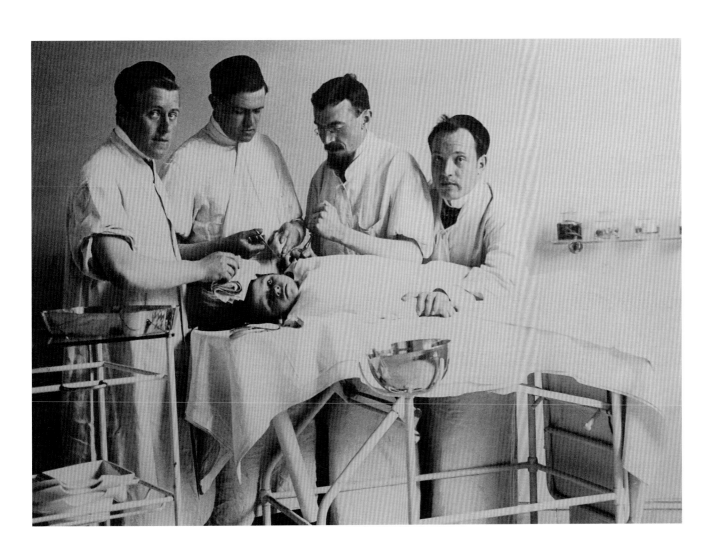

## 24
## Tuberculosis of the Larynx:
## Examination for This Deadly Complication
### Gelatin Silver Print, 9 by 12 inches
### Havana, Cuba
### circa 1895

This physician examines the throat of a tuberculosis patient to identify laryngeal tubercles. One of the dreaded late complications of tuberculosis was its spread to the larynx. By continually discharging into the main bronchial pathways laryngeal tubercles rapidly seeded the disease through both lungs. Indeed, the symptoms of hoarseness, difficulty swallowing, and throat pain usually heralded a swift downhill course with death finally resulting from pulmonary tuberculosis. This photograph was taken in the hospital throat room in a tuberculosis clinic in Havana, Cuba. It is identified as the "Samoza Dispensary." The physician wears a head mirror with a gas lamp for illumination. The protective glass partition between the physician and patient marks the critical recognition of airborne contagion by tuberculosis. Laryngeal tuberculosis presents as tuberculin ulcers or nodules and was first identified in the early nineteenth century. Tuberculosis specialists such as Broussais, Laënnec, Andrail, Trousseau and others attempted to differentiate the various types of laryngeal tuberculosis. However, as the larynx was inaccessible to the physician's direct observation, the study and diagnosis of laryngeal lesions remained guesswork in the living patient. Only postmortem observation of the throat could give an accurate diagnosis. In 1854, singing teacher, Manuel Garcia (1805-1906), invented the modern laryngoscope to observe the vocal cords. Viennese physician, Ludwig Turck, M.D. (1810-1868), attempted to use the scope to view the larynx but lacked sufficient reflected light. Johann Czermak, M.D. (1828-1873) invented the headband mirror to use with the laryngoscope, making clinical use of the instrument feasible. As in the case of the discovery of anesthesia both physicians fought their entire professional careers over the question of who was the first to accurately diagnose laryngeal lesions. Once easily viewed the laryngeal lesions could be treated. In the nineteenth century treatment of the disease involved nearly every drug that could be applied to the area by spray, inhalation, injection, rubbing, etc. Electrocauterization and surgery were also attempted. None of these modalities, however, altered the fatal course of the disease. Contracting laryngeal tuberculosis was a death sentence until the twentieth century.

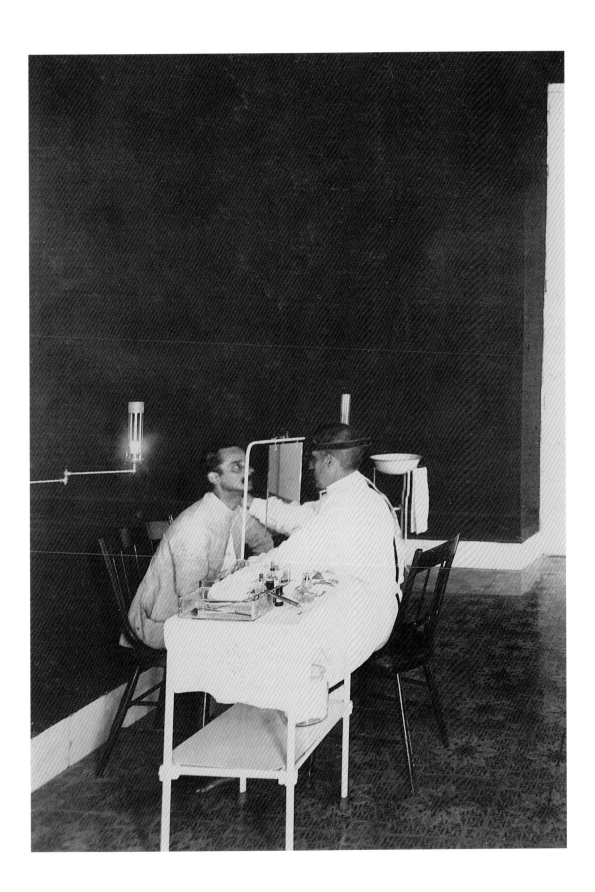

## 25
## WAITING OUT THE PNEUMONIA CRISIS
### SILVER PRINT, 5 BY 7 INCHES
### CIRCA 1895

In the pre-antibiotic era, pneumonia was a dreaded killer of the young and a welcomed friend of the very old. Prior to the specific therapies and antibiotics of the twentieth century many patients were better off if their disease ran its natural course. Numerous bacteria cause pneumonia and depending on the pathogenicity of the bacteria the survival rate varied. Untreated lobar pneumonia had a 30% mortality. One of the most common infections was pneumococcal pneumonia. It had a predictable, natural course and included the symptoms of dyspnea, blood tinged sputum, pleuritic pain, fever and chills. After 7 to 10 days a "crisis" occurred consisting of sweating with defervescence and spontaneous resolution. During much of the nineteenth century physicians attempted to intervene in the course of the disease with drastic therapies and medications. Blood letting was commonly used in lung disease 'to relieve congestion'; mercury, opium, alcohol and other dangerous drugs were used in an attempt to rally the patient. Some of these drugs suppress respiration. Alternative medical practitioners, such as homeopaths, with their extremely dilute medications, provided little intervention and thus seemed to help patients as the disease ran its course. Once astute physicians realized they could not safely alter the course of the disease, they offered supportive therapy, fluids, blankets and watchful waiting. Thus doing nothing was often the best therapy. By the turn of the century distrust of doctors was almost a thing of the past. This photograph is common of many similar images of physicians, nurses and the family about the bedside. Many times comments such as "she will be better" were attached to the photograph. The implication being the physicians knew what they were doing, and had confidence in the outcome. It must be noted, pneumonia is still a deadly disease especially when combined with influenza. In the 1990s, in this combination it was the sixth leading cause of death in the United States.

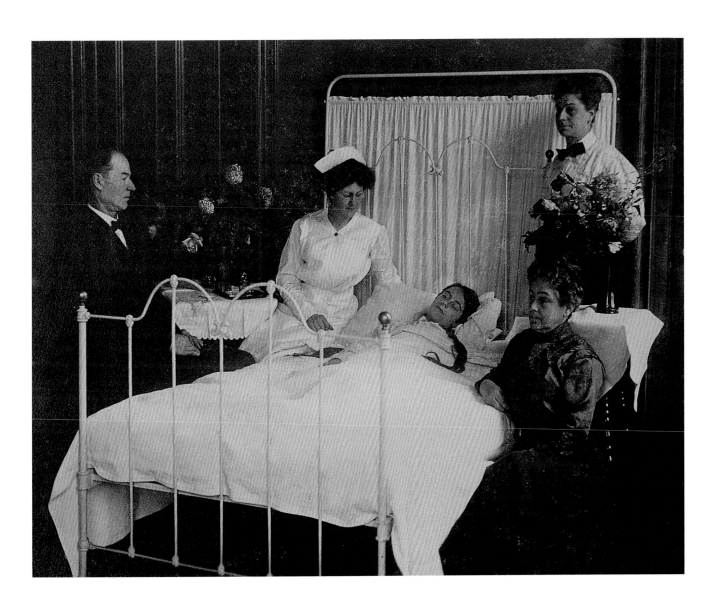

# BIBLIOGRAPHY

Bordley III, James, M.D., and A. Harvey McGehee, M.D. *Two Centuries of American Medicine: 1776-1976*. W.B. Saunders Co.: Philadelphia, Pennsylvania, 1976.

Brandt, Allan M. *No Magic Bullet: A Social History of Venereal Disease in the United States Since 1880*. Oxford University Press: New York, New York, 1985.

Brieger, Gert H. *Medical America in the Nineteenth Century: Readings from the Literature*. Johns Hopkins Press: Baltimore, Maryland, 1972.

Burns, Stanley B., M.D., and Richard Glenner, D.D.S. et al. *The American Dentist: A Pictorial History with a Presentation of Early Dental Photography in America*. Pictorial Histories Publishing Co.: Missoula, MT, 1990.

Burns, Stanley B., M.D., and Ira M. Rutkow, M.D. *American Surgery: An Illustrated History*. Lippincott-Raven Publishers: Philadelphia, PA, 1998.

Burns, Stanley B., M.D. *Early Medical Photography in America: 1839-1883*. The Burns Archive: New York, NY, 1983.

Burns, Stanley B., M.D., and Sherwin Nuland, M.D. et al. *The Face of Mercy: A Photographic History of Medicine at War*. Random House: New York, NY, 1993.

Burns, Stanley B., M.D., and Joel-Peter Witkin, et al. *Harm's Way: Lust & Madness, Murder & Mayhem*. Twin Palms Publishers: Santa Fe, New Mexico, 1994.

Burns, Stanley B., M.D., and Joel-Peter Witkin, et al. *Masterpieces of Medical Photography: Selections From The Burns Archive*. Twelvetrees Press: Pasadena, CA 1987.

Burns, Stanley B., M.D., *A Morning's Work: Medical Photographs from The Burns Archive & Collection 1843-1939*. Twin Palms Publishers: Santa Fe, New Mexico, 1998.

Burns, Stanley B., M.D., and Jacques Gasser, M.D. *Photographie et Médecine 1840-1880*. Insitut universitaire d'histoire de la santé publique: Lausanne, Switzerland, 1991.

Burns, Stanley B., M.D. *Sleeping Beauty: Memorial Photography in America*. TwelveTrees Press: Altadena, California, 1990.

Burns, Stanley B., M.D. and Elizabeth A. Burns. *Sleeping Beauty II: Grief, Bereavement and The Family in Medical Photography, American & European Traditions*. Burns Archive Press: New York, NY, 2002.

Clarke, Edward H., M.D. et al. *A Century of American Medicine: 1776-1876*. Burt Franklin: New York, NY, 1876.

Conway, Herbert, M.D. and Richard Stark, M.D. *Plastic Surgery at the New York Hospital One Hundred Years Ago*. Paul B. Hoeber, Inc.: New York, NY, 1953.

Cummins, S. Lyle, M.D. *Tuberculosis in History: From the 17th Century to our Times*. Bailliere, Tindall and Cox: London, 1949.

Davis, Loyal. *Fifty Years of Surgical Progress: 1905-1955*. Franklin H. Martin Memorial Foundation: Chicago, Illinois, 1955.

Dieffenbach, William H. *Hydrotherapy: A Brief Therapy of the Practical Value of Water in Disease for Students and Practicians of Medicine*. Rebman Co.: New York, NY, 1909.

Donahue, M. Patricia. *Nursing: The Finest Art*. Mosby: St. Louis, Missouri, 1996.

Duffy, John. *The Healers: A History of American Medicine*. University of Illinois Press: Urbana, Illinois, 1976.

Dubos, Rene and Jean. *The White Plague: Tuberculosis, Man and Society*. Little Brown and Company: Boston, MA, 1952.

Editors. *Harrison's Principles of Internal Medicine, Thirteenth Edition*. McGraw Hill: Health Professionals Division, 1994.

Fee, Elizabeth and Daniel M. Fox. *AIDS: The Burdens of History*. University of California Press: Berkeley, California, 1988.

Frizot, Michel. *The New History of Photograph.*, Könemann Verlagsgesellschaft mbH: Koln, Germany, 1998.

Fye, W. Bruce, M.D. *The Development of American Physiology: Scientific Medicine in the Nineteenth Century*. Johns Hopkins University Press: Baltimore, Maryland, 1987.

Fye, W. Bruce. M.D. *American Cardiology: The History of a Specialty and Its College*. Johns Hopkins University Press: Baltimore, Maryland, 1996.

Garrison, Fielding H. M.D. *An Introduction to the History of Medicine. With Medical Chronology, Suggestions for Study and Bibliographic Data*. W.B. Saunders Co.: Philadelphia, Pennsylvania, 1913.

Gevitz, Norman. *The DO's: Osteopathic Medicine in America*. Johns Hopkins University Press: Baltimore, MD, 1982.

Gorin, George. *History of Ophthalmology*. Publish or Perish, Inc.: Wilmington, Delaware, 1982.

Hechtlinger, Adelaide. *The Great Patent Medicine Era or Without Benefit of Doctor*. Grosset & Dunlap, Inc.: New York, NY, 1970.

Hopkins, Donald R. *Princes and Peasants: Smallpox in History*. University of Chicago Press: Chicago and London, 1983.

Hurwitz, Alfred, M.D. and George Degenshein, M.D. *Milestones in Modern Surgery*. Hoeber-Harper, New York, NY, 1958.

Johnson, Stephen L. *The History of Cardiac Surgery: 1896-1955*. Johns Hopkins Press: Baltimore, Maryland, 1970.

Keen, William W. M.D. *Surgery; Its Principles and Practice, by Various Authors*. W.B. Saunders Co.: Philadelphia, PA, 1908.

Kelly, Howard and Walter Burrage. *Dictionary of American Medical Biography*. D. Appleton and Co.: New York, NY, 1928.

Kevles, Bettyann Holtzmann. *Naked to the Bone: Medical Imaging in the Twentieth Century*. Helix Books, Addison Wesley: Reading, Massachusetts, 1997.

Kevorkian, Jack, M.D. *The Story of Dissection*. Philosophical Library: New York, NY, 1959.

Kiple, Kenneth F. *The Cambridge World History of Human Disease*. Cambridge University Press: New York, NY, 1993.

Leibowitz, J.O. *The History of Coronary Heart Disease*. Wellcome Institute of the History of Medicine: London, 1970.

Levinson, Abraham, M.D. *Pioneers of Pediatrics*. Froben Press: New York, NY, 1936.

Lieberman, Phillip, M.D. and Michael Blaiss, M.D. *Atlas of Allergic Diseases*. Current Medicine, Inc.: Philadelphia, PA, 2002.

Lopate, Carol. *Women in Medicine*. Johns Hopkins Press: Baltimore, Maryland, 1968.

Lyons, Albert S., M.D. and J.S. Petrucelli II, M.D. *Medicine: An Illustrated History*. Harry N. Abrams, Inc.: New York, NY, 1978.

Margotta, Roberto. *The Story of Medicine*. Golden Press: New

# BIBLIOGRAPHY

Bordley III, James, M.D., and A. Harvey McGehee, M.D. *Two Centuries of American Medicine: 1776-1976*. W.B. Saunders Co.: Philadelphia, Pennsylvania, 1976.

Brandt, Allan M. *No Magic Bullet: A Social History of Venereal Disease in the United States Since 1880*. Oxford University Press: New York, New York, 1985.

Brieger, Gert H. *Medical America in the Nineteenth Century: Readings from the Literature*. Johns Hopkins Press: Baltimore, Maryland, 1972.

Burns, Stanley B., M.D., and Richard Glenner, D.D.S. et al. *The American Dentist: A Pictorial History with a Presentation of Early Dental Photography in America*. Pictorial Histories Publishing Co.: Missoula, MT, 1990.

Burns, Stanley B., M.D., and Ira M. Rutkow, M.D. *American Surgery: An Illustrated History*. Lippincott-Raven Publishers: Philadelphia, PA, 1998.

Burns, Stanley B., M.D. *Early Medical Photography in America: 1839-1883*. The Burns Archive: New York, NY, 1983.

Burns, Stanley B., M.D., and Sherwin Nuland, M.D. et al. *The Face of Mercy: A Photographic History of Medicine at War*. Random House: New York, NY, 1993.

Burns, Stanley B., M.D., and Joel-Peter Witkin, et al. *Harm's Way: Lust & Madness, Murder & Mayhem*. Twin Palms Publishers: Santa Fe, New Mexico, 1994.

Burns, Stanley B., M.D., and Joel-Peter Witkin, et al. *Masterpieces of Medical Photography: Selections From The Burns Archive*. Twelvetrees Press: Pasadena, CA 1987.

Burns, Stanley B., M.D., *A Morning's Work: Medical Photographs from The Burns Archive & Collection 1843-1939*. Twin Palms Publishers: Santa Fe, New Mexico, 1998.

Burns, Stanley B., M.D., and Jacques Gasser, M.D. *Photographie et Médecine 1840-1880*. Insitut universitaire d'histoire de la santé publique: Lausanne, Switzerland, 1991.

Burns, Stanley B., M.D. *Sleeping Beauty: Memorial Photography in America*. TwelveTrees Press: Altadena, California, 1990.

Burns, Stanley B., M.D. and Elizabeth A. Burns. *Sleeping Beauty II: Grief, Bereavement and The Family in Medical Photography, American & European Traditions*. Burns Archive Press: New York, NY, 2002.

Clarke, Edward H., M.D. et al. *A Century of American Medicine: 1776-1876*. Burt Franklin: New York, NY, 1876.

Conway, Herbert, M.D. and Richard Stark, M.D. *Plastic Surgery at the New York Hospital One Hundred Years Ago*. Paul B. Hoeber, Inc.: New York, NY, 1953.

Cummins, S. Lyle, M.D. *Tuberculosis in History: From the 17th Century to our Times*. Bailliere, Tindall and Cox: London, 1949.

Davis, Loyal. *Fifty Years of Surgical Progress: 1905-1955*. Franklin H. Martin Memorial Foundation: Chicago, Illinois, 1955.

Dieffenbach, William H. *Hydrotherapy: A Brief Therapy of the Practical Value of Water in Disease for Students and Practicians of Medicine*. Rebman Co.: New York, NY, 1909.

Donahue, M. Patricia. *Nursing: The Finest Art*. Mosby: St. Louis, Missouri, 1996.

Duffy, John. *The Healers: A History of American Medicine*. University of Illinois Press: Urbana, Illinois, 1976.

Dubos, Rene and Jean. *The White Plague: Tuberculosis, Man and*

# PHOTOGRAPHIC TERMS

## HARD IMAGES

**Daguerreotype:**
The daguerreotype, the first practical form of photography, was presented to the world in 1839 by Frenchman, Louis J.M. Daguerre. It was popular between 1839-1860. It consisted of an image developed on a polished, silver coated, copper plate. This fragile surface made it necessary to protect the plate behind a glass cover and within a special case. Daguerreotypes and ambrotypes were both produced in standard sizes that had a direct relation to the plate size used in the camera.

**Ambrotype:**
This form of photography was popular between 1854-1865. The ambrotype was a process using silver sensitive emulsion placed on glass. Like the daguerreotype the surface was fragile and the image was cased.

**Tintype:**
Although most popular between 1858-1890, tintypes, patented in 1856, were produced as a novelty until about 1940. In the tintype process the silver emulsion was affixed to a thin sheet of iron. This surface was not fragile and tintypes could even be sent through the mail. The term "tintype" comes from the use of tin snips to cut the large sheets of iron.

## PAPER PRINTS

The calotype, the first type of paper print made from a paper negative, was invented in 1841. The process was not used in America. In 1851, the collodion wet plate process was developed using glass negatives. The photographic glass negative had to be wet when inserted into the camera and immediately developed while still wet. The paper albumen print was its most popular form. In 1871, Englishman Richard Maddox, MD developed the gelatin based silver print, known as the dry plate process. By the late 1870s instantaneous stop action photographs were possible. Photographs were usually taken by professionals or serious amateurs until 1888 when Kodak introduced roll film with a special camera that allowed anyone to take a photograph. The age of amateur photography began and physicians began to personally document their lives and patients.

**Carte de Visite:**
Most popular between 1860-1880, the CdV was a $2^1/_4$ by $3^1/_2$ inch paper print pasted onto a card $2^1/_2$ by 4 inches. It was this style photograph that necessitated the creation of the photograph album, so the public could easily compile cards of relatives or celebrities.

**Cabinet Card:**
Popular between 1875-1895, the cabinet card is a 4 by $5^1/_2$ inch print pasted on a $4^1/_4$ by $6^1/_2$ inch card. Cabinet cards were also assembled in albums.

**Stereoview:**
Popular from 1850-1930, the stereoview encompassed all the different photographic processes. It consisted of two images each about 3 by $3^1/_2$ taken with a special twin-lens camera. The prints were mounted side by side on a cardboard about $3^1/_2$ by 7 inches. The card was inserted into a stereoscope viewer, which created a 3D effect and gave the viewer the illusion of actually viewing the scene. This three dimensional effect was useful in teaching medical subjects.

**Albumen Print:**
Popular 1850s-1880, the albumen print was a sharp, detailed paper print produced by the wet plate process. An egg white based emulsion was the key to this process, hence the name 'albumen' print.

**Gelatin-Silver Print & other Silver Print Processes:**
Popular in various forms from 1880 to today.

# DEDICATION

Many physicians who treated and investigated tuberculosis contracted and succumbed to the disease. The list is voluminous and contains many medical luminaries including Dr. Rene Laënnec, inventor of the stethoscope. The sacrifices made by physicians for the advancement of medicine are legendary. Those who died or were mutilated in the development of radiology are well known but the specialists and conquerors fighting tuberculosis have never been fully appreciated. To these selfless individuals, I dedicate this work.

# ACKNOWLEDGEMENTS

First and foremost I would like to thank my family who are integral parts of the Burns Archive. They have assisted me, tirelessly, in preparing this historic compilation. My wife, Sara, helps with collecting, cataloging and archiving the collection, and directs the stock photography use of the material. More importantly she serves as my sounding board and editor helping to clarify my ideas. My daughter, Elizabeth, designed and directed the entire production of these volumes from their conception to the final product.

I am most grateful to Saul G. Hornik, MS, RPh, medical marketing consultant. It was his enthusiasm and recognition of the educational importance of my medical, photographic collection, together with his tireless work that made this publication a reality. I give my thanks to Eric Malter, President of MD Communications, for his support of this project. I also wish to express my sincere appreciation to Christopher J. Carney, Director of Training Services of GlaxoSmithKline for understanding the educational value in using the visual history of the past as a foundation for the future.

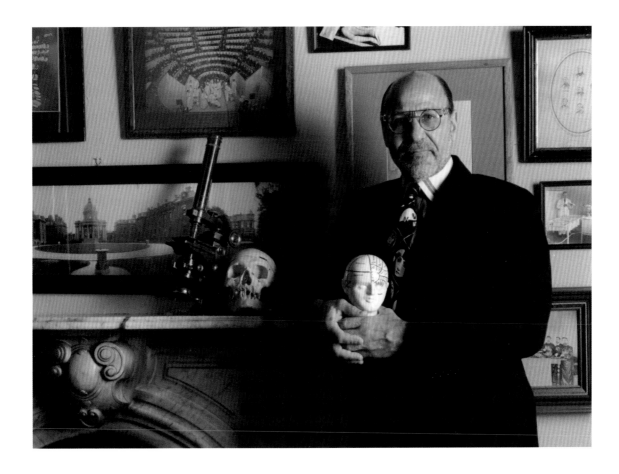

# Stanley B. Burns, M.D., F.A.C.S.

Stanley B. Burns, M.D., F.A.C.S., a practicing New York City ophthalmic surgeon, is also an internationally distinguished photographic historian, author, curator and collector. His collection, started in 1975, is considered to be the most comprehensive private, early, historic photograph collection in the world. Contained within this archive of over 700,000 vintage prints is the finest and most comprehensive compilation of early medical photographs, consisting of 50,000 images taken between 1840 and 1940. These medical photographs have been showcased in countless publications, films and museum exhibitions. France's Channel Plus prepared a documentary on his work as part of the *Great Collectors of the World Series*. Dr. Burns has been an active medical historian since 1970. From 1979-81, he was President of the Medical Archivist of New York State. He has been a member of the medical history departments of The Albert Einstein College of Medicine and The State University of New York, Medical College at Stony Brook; Curator of photographic archives at both The Israeli Institute on The History of Medicine (1978-1993) and The Museum of The Foundation of The American Academy of Ophthalmology. Currently, he is a contributing editor for five specialty medical journals. The Burns Archive, his stock photography and publishing entity, is a valuable photographic resource for both researchers and the media. Using his unique collection Dr. Burns has written ten award winning, photo-history books, hundreds of articles and curated dozens of exhibitions. His film company, Black Mirror Films, produced *Death in America*, an award willing documentary on the history of death practices in America. He is currently working on several medical exhibitions and books, as well as photographic history books on criminology, Judaica, Germans in WW II and African Americans. He can be reached through his web site www.burnsarchive.com.

## OTHER BOOKS

*Sleeping Beauty II: Grief, Bereavement and The Family in Memorial Photography, American & European Traditions*

*A Mornings Work: Medical Photographs from The Burns Archive & Collection, 1843-1939*

*Forgotten Marriage: The Painted Tintype & The Decorative Frame 1860-1910, A Lost Chapter in American Portraiture*

*American Surgery: An Illustrated History*
co-author: Ira M. Rutkow, M.D.

*Harm's Way: Lust & Madness, Murder & Mayhem*
co-authors: Joel-Peter Witkin, et al

*The Face of Mercy: A Photographic History of Medicine at War*
co-authors: Matthew Naythons, M.D. and Sherwin Nuland, M.D.

*Photographie et Médecine 1840-1880*
co-author: Jacques Gasser, M.D.

*Sleeping Beauty: Memorial Photography in America*

*The American Dentist: A Pictorial History*
co-authors: Richard Glenner, D.D.S. and Audrey Davis, PhD.

*Masterpieces of Medical Photography: Selections From The Burns Archive*
co-author: Joel-Peter Witkin

*Early Medical Photography in America: 1839-1883*

THE BURNS ARCHIVE PRESS
140 EAST 38TH STREET • NEW YORK, N.Y. 10016
TEL: 212-889-1938 • FAX: 212-481-9113 • WWW.BURNSARCHIVE.COM